Health Unit
COORDINATING

formerly Unit Secretary

CERTIFICATION REVIEW

Fifth Edition

Health Unit COORDINATING

formerly Unit Secretary

CERTIFICATION REVIEW

Myrna LaFleur Brooks, RN, BEd, CHUC
Founding President, National Association of Health Unit Coordinators
Faculty Emeritus, Maricopa County Community College District
Phoenix, Arizona

Elaine A. Gillingham, AAS, BA, CHUC
Director, Health Unit Coordinator Program
GateWay Community College
Phoenix, Arizona

SAUNDERS

An Imprint of Elsevier

SAUNDERS
An Imprint of Elsevier

11830 Westline Industrial Drive
St. Louis, Missouri 63146

NOTICE

Medicine is an ever-changing field. Standard safety precautions must be followed, but as new research and clinical experience broaden our knowledge, changes in treatment and drug therapy may become necessary or appropriate. Readers are advised to check the most current product information provided by the manufacturer of each drug to be administered to verify the recommended dose, the method and duration of administration, and contraindications. It is the responsibility of the licensed prescriber, relying on experience and knowledge of the patient, to determine dosages and the best treatment for each individual patient. Neither the publisher nor the author assumes any liability for any injury and/or damage to persons or property arising from this publication.

Previous editions copyrighted 1998, 1993, 1986, 1979

ISBN-13: 978-0-7216-0100-7
ISBN-10: 0-7216-0100-6

Executive Editor: Adrianne Cochran
Developmental Editors: Helaine Tobin, Rose Foltz
Publishing Services Manager: Pat Joiner
Designer: Kathi Gosche

Printed in the United States of America

Last digit is the print number: 9 8 7 6 5 4

PREFACE

This most recent edition of *Health Unit Coordinating Certification Review* prepares health unit coordinators to sit for the certification exam sponsored by the National Association of Health Unit Coordinators. As in the four previous editions, this textbook is designed to be a self-assessment of knowledge and practice of health unit coordinating. It is intended to assist you in reviewing and assessing your knowledge of material covered in the fifth edition of *Health Unit Coordinating*. Preparing to sit for a certification exam requires one to address a large volume of material. Using the self-assessment review book will assist you in determining what you already know and what you need to learn. This awareness should ease the preparation process and assist you in making the best use of your time.

The book consists of sample multiple choice test questions, similar in style to those used on the national exam. The questions correspond with the chapters of *Health Unit Coordinating*, 5th edition. The correct answer for each question and the rationale for the answer are provided. Each answer is followed by a reference page number in *Health Unit Coordinating*, 5th edition, which guides you to more information on the subject matter as needed.

This edition has been expanded to include questions about the latest changes in health care technology and the Health Insurance Portability and Accountability Act (HIPAA) Privacy Rule, as well as the latest in health unit coordinating practice. It also includes a final section that presents employment-related situation questions. This portion deals with employment situations and decision-making using the techniques included in *Health Unit Coordinating*, 5th edition. A mock exam is included, consisting of 120 questions similar to those you will see when taking the national certification exam. This mock exam is provided so you can test yourself, gain insight, and better prepare to take the national certification exam.

If you are reading this you have probably already decided to sit for the certification exam for health unit coordinators. Certification is a systematic process that recognizes and publicly attests to a person's mastery of knowledge and achievement of skills in a particular specialty. It is a voluntary process. The National Association of Health Unit Coordinators offered the first exam in 1983.

Recertification is now available by retaking the NAHUC certification exam every 3 years, or by accumulating 36 CMUs (continuing maintenance units) over a 3-year period. By recertifying, you will show a continued competence to practice in the health unit coordinator field.

As more demands are being placed on the health care industry, hiring professional, certified employees will assist institutions in meeting production demands. Being certified in your field may very well expand your opportunity for employment, for mobility, and possibly for career advancement. We compliment you on your decision to sit for the exam and wish you success in this endeavor.

Myrna LaFleur Brooks and Elaine A. Gillingham

TIPS FOR TEST TAKING

1. Preparation for the test is vital. Plan for quality study time at a desk or wherever you feel comfortable. Choose a quiet place, perhaps with your choice of background music. An environment without interruptions is best.

2. The exam is an objective exam, sometimes referred to as a multiple-choice exam. Each question has a stem, the main portion of the question, and four options that either complete the statement or answer the question. There is one correct answer and three plausible distracters. The distracters are not meant to trick you but they may distract you from the correct answer.

3. Read each stem and each option as if it were a separate true-false statement. Look for key words in the stem such as *first, most important, left* or *right, not, except,* and so forth.

4. Read all options carefully before selecting the correct answer. Do not read more into the question.

5. Sometimes the option that has the most words is correct. Item writers are aware of this and may try to avoid giving this as a clue.

6. The number or letter of the correct answer may be the same as several preceding it. When choosing your answer, do not be tempted to vary your answer for this reason.

7. An option may be chosen on impulse and then changed on review. Avoid this. Studies have shown that the first answer that comes to mind is usually right.

8. Do not spend more than a minute or two on a question. If you are having difficulty selecting an answer, note that you did not answer the question, move on to the next, and then return to the unanswered questions when you have completed the exam. Subsequent questions may give you clues to the correct answer.

9. Take time to read the test-taking directions, and then follow them carefully. Failure to do so may result in your correct answer being scored by the computer program as a wrong answer. If, for example, when using a touch-screen computer, you select an answer above or below the correct answer you meant to select, the computer program will read it as an incorrect answer. Do not hesitate to ask questions if you do not know how to proceed.

10. Answer all questions, because the scoring is the same whether you answer incorrectly or not at all, and you may select the correct answer by chance.

11. Prepare yourself mentally for the exam. Try positive mental imagery. Imagine yourself taking the test with the confidence that you are selecting the correct answers. Imagine yourself receiving a passing score. Having positive thoughts about your ability to perform can affect your actual performance.

12. Get plenty of rest the night before the exam.

CONTENTS

Orientation to Hospitals, Medical Centers, and Health Care

Health Unit Coordinating

An Allied Health Career

1. You are a health unit coordinator and want to make yourself as marketable as possible; you would:
   a. exaggerate your work experience on your resume
   b. be especially nice to the nurse managers
   c. work as much overtime as possible
   d. become certified

2. To be "certified" means that the health unit coordinator has:
   a. completed an educational program at a community college
   b. worked more than 300 hours in an accredited hospital
   c. passed an examination sponsored by the National Association of Health Unit Coordinators
   d. earned an associate degree in health unit coordinating

3. The health unit coordinator would refer which of the following tasks to the nurse:
   a. communicate a doctor's order to the responsible hospital departments
   b. inform a visitor of hospital rules and patient location
   c. answer the nursing unit telephone
   d. answer a patient's questions regarding test results

4. Which of the following items of information would be found in the policy and procedure manual?
   a. job descriptions
   b. physician phone numbers
   c. patient census
   d. health record codes

5. National guidelines serving as a model of performance by which health unit coordinators shall conduct their actions are known as a:
   a. standard of practice
   b. code of ethics
   c. job description
   d. policy manual

6. Which of the following is considered a clinical task?
   a. answering a patient's call on the intercom
   b. transcribing doctor's orders
   c. calling in or receiving lab results
   d. assisting a patient to the bathroom

7. Dr. Smith is performing an LP procedure in the examining room. You hear a page for Dr. Smith and realize the page cannot be heard in the exam room. Your most appropriate action is to:
   a. ignore the page, knowing the operator will probably take the message
   b. ask the operator to transfer the call to the exam room
   c. explain to the operator that the doctor is busy and can be reached later
   d. take the message and deliver it to the doctor

☑ **ANSWERS AND RATIONALE**

1. **(d)** Certification would provide credibility and would make you more marketable. pp. 6, 7

> *pp. 6, 7*, refers to the page number in *Health Unit Coordinating*, 5th edition, where you can find more information on the subject of the question. Using this text with the review book is a must to develop the knowledge base necessary for successfully completing the examination.

2. **(c)** To be a certified health unit coordinator one must sit for and pass the National Certification Exam. pp. 6, 7

> The National Certification Program is sponsored by the National Health Unit Coordinator Certification Board, which is a part of the National Association of Health Unit Coordinators. The Association was established in 1980 in Phoenix, Arizona. The first certification examination was offered in 1983.

3. **(d)** The patient's doctor or nurse would answer questions regarding test results. pp. 7–9
4. **(a)** Job descriptions as well as guidelines for practice and hospital regulations would be addressed in the policy and procedure manual. pp. 4, 10
5. **(a)** The standard of practice is established by the professional association to be used as a standard nationwide. p. 5
6. **(d)** Assisting a patient to the restroom is a clinical task. p. 3
7. **(d)** Take the message and deliver it to the doctor. The HUC manages and performs the receptionist role for a nursing unit and performs the telephone communications for the nursing unit. pp. 7–9

> LP is the abbreviation for lumbar puncture, a procedure used to remove cerebrospinal fluid from the spinal canal.

8. Recertification is a requirement by NAHUC to:
   a. make money for the association
   b. offset the cost of certification materials
   c. force review of what HUCs once learned
   d. ensure that certified HUCs stay current in their field of practice

9. To copy a patient's chart for a physician, you would follow the procedure as described in the:
   a. HUC job description
   b. health record guide
   c. policy and procedure manual
   d. disaster manual

10. The first organizational meeting for the Health Unit Coordinator Association was held in:
    a. Toledo
    b. Phoenix
    c. Chicago
    d. Minneapolis

11. The overall job of the health unit coordinator is to coordinate and perform:
    a. clinical tasks for the nursing unit
    b. non-clinical tasks for the nursing unit
    c. all tasks requested by the head nurse
    d. both clinical and non-clinical tasks for the nursing unit

12. A nurse asks you to perform a task that you have not been trained for. You do not feel comfortable in performing this task. You would:
    a. find the procedure for performing the task in the policy and procedure manual and follow it
    b. call one of the other HUCs who has been cross-trained and ask him or her how to do the task
    c. do the task and hope you do it correctly
    d. inform the nurse that you have not been trained to do that task and that you do not feel comfortable in doing it until you have received training

13. Independent transcription may be described as:
    a. the nurse caring for the patient is responsible for transcribing the physician's orders; cosignature is not required
    b. the HUC assumes full responsibility for transcription of physician's orders; cosignature by a nurse is not required
    c. the charge nurse transcribes the physician's orders; cosignature of the nurse caring for the patient is required
    d. the HUC assumes full responsibility for the transcription of the physician's orders; cosignature of the RN is required

14. National Health Unit Coordinator day is on:
    a. July 1
    b. August 23
    c. January 20
    d. May 23

15. Which of the following is an advantage for the health unit coordinator to be a member of NAHUC:
    a. professional representation
    b. tuition reimbursement
    c. union grievance process available
    d. guaranteed higher pay

☑ *ANSWERS AND RATIONALE*

8. **(d)** Recertification is a process of testifying to or endorsing that a person has met certain standards. pp. 4, 7
9. **(c)** The policy and procedure manual contains guidelines for practice and hospital regulations and procedures. p. 4
10. **(b)** The first organizational meeting for the National Association of Health Unit Coordinators was held in Phoenix, Arizona on August 23, 1980. p. 5
11. **(b)** The overall job of the health unit coordinator is to coordinate and perform the non-clinical tasks for the nursing unit. p. 4

> Throughout the text, the most up-to-date term, *health unit coordinator*, is used instead of "unit secretary" or "unit clerk."

12. **(d)** You should not perform tasks that you have not been trained to do. p. 10
13. **(b)** The HUC assumes full responsibility for transcription of doctors' orders; therefore, cosignature by the nurse is not required. p. 3
14. **(b)** National Health Unit Coordinator day is on August 23rd. p. 5
15. **(a)** Professional representation is an advantage of being a member of NAHUC. p. 7

> For information on joining NAHUC, The National Association for Health Unit Coordinators, or to obtain copies of the Standards of Practice and Education or the Code of Ethics, call 1-888-22-NAHUC (62482) (or locally 815-633-4351); fax: 815-633-4438; visit the web site: www.nahuc.org; e-mail: office@nahuc.org, or write to:
> National Association of Health Unit Coordinators
> 1947 Madron Road
> Rockford, IL 61107

Health Care Today

1. The hospital where you work is preparing for a visit from JCAHO. The purpose of this visit is so the hospital may receive:
   a. capitation
   b. quality assurance
   c. accreditation
   d. certification

2. Managed care was created because:
   a. doctors were not treating patients appropriately
   b. insurance companies were making too much money
   c. health care costs were increasing
   d. doctors were not ordering the needed tests

3. DRGs are:
   a. discounted registered generic medications
   b. drug restrictions for geriatrics
   c. drug regulated growth
   d. diagnosis-related groups

4. "Capitation" is a term currently used in health care that means:
   a. hospitals have a limit on the number of patients who can be admitted per year
   b. a payment method whereby the provider of care receives a set dollar amount per patient regardless of services provided.
   c. only a certain number of hospitals are approved to operate within a given population
   d. hospitals are limited in how much money is spent on new equipment per year

5. Accreditation means that the hospital has:
   a. met an official standard
   b. a license to operate
   c. approval from the state department of health
   d. approval from a medical association

6. Which of the following departments of the hospital records and analyzes incidents that occur involving patients?
   a. security
   b. quality assurance
   c. human resources
   d. public relations

7. Which of the following is in direct charge of the hospital?
   a. medical staff
   b. hospital CEO
   c. hospital CFO
   d. hospital COO

8. Which of the following would the CEO report to?
   a. medical staff
   b. vice president of nursing
   c. governing board
   d. hospital COO

9. Which of the following is a responsibility of the governing board?
   a. establishing policies
   b. purchasing hospital supplies
   c. performing employee evaluations
   d. supervising quality patient care

☑ *Answers And Rationale*

1. **(c)** JCAHO (Joint Commission on Accreditation of Healthcare Organizations) is the agency that accredits hospitals as well as other health care facilities. p. 18

2. **(c)** Managed care was created because of increasing costs of health care; insurance companies were going bankrupt. p. 24

3. **(d)** DRG stands for diagnosis-related groups, which provide prospective payment for hospital services based on the patient's admitting diagnosis and thereby reduces the overall cost. pp. 15, 24

4. **(b)** Capitation is a payment method whereby the providers of care receive a set dollar amount per patient regardless of services rendered. pp. 14, 24

5. **(a)** Accreditation means the hospital has met an official standard such as accreditation from JCAHO. Accreditation is voluntary. A license to operate is required and usually is granted by the State Department of Health Services. pp. 14, 18

6. **(b)** Quality assurance provides information to various departments within the hospital for the purpose of helping those departments provide quality care. pp. 21, 22

7. **(b)** The chief executive officer (CEO) is in direct charge of the hospital. p. 18

8. **(c)** The hospital CEO is responsible to the governing board. p. XXX

9. **(a)** The governing board would have the responsibility of establishing policies. p. 18

10. A doctor wishing to join the medical staff of a hospital must be approved by the:
    a. medical staff
    b. governing board
    c. hospital CEO
    d. vice president of nursing

11. A doctor who admits patients to the hospital is known as a/an:
    a. resident physician
    b. attending physician
    c. specialist physician
    d. intern physician

12. Which of the following is the title for a medical school graduate gaining hospital experience?
    a. clinical clerk
    b. osteopath
    c. resident
    d. specialist

13. The person within the hospital who coordinates the patient's care with the insurance companies is the:
    a. case manager
    b. unit manager
    c. house officer
    d. vice president of nursing

14. A specialist in glandular diseases is called a/an:
    a. allergist
    b. endocrinologist
    c. neonatologist
    d. radiologist

15. A radiologist is employed by which of the following hospital departments?
    a. cardiovascular studies
    b. electroencephalography
    c. diagnostic imaging
    d. respiratory care

16. Diagnostic studies related to brain-wave disorders are performed in which of the following departments?
    a. neurodiagnostics
    b. endoscopy
    c. physical therapy
    d. diagnostic imaging

17. Personnel from which of the following departments assist in maintaining a patient on a ventilator?
    a. endoscopy
    b. physical therapy
    c. respiratory care
    d. diagnostic imaging

18. The purpose of the radiation oncology department is to:
    a. take x-rays
    b. treat cancerous growths
    c. make diagnoses through the use of a scanner
    d. perform lung function tests

19. On discharge, the patient's record is coded and then stored for future retrieval or for research. The department responsible for this is:
    a. personnel
    b. business office
    c. health records
    d. admitting

20. The hospital department that performs diagnostic procedures on body specimens, such as tissue, and also performs autopsies is:
    a. pulmonary function
    b. pathology
    c. endoscopy
    d. gastroenterology

21. Visual examinations of hollow organs or body cavities are performed by which of the following departments?
    a. electroencephalography
    b. physical medicine
    c. oncology
    d. endoscopy

22. A visitor is insisting, in a loud and angry voice, to see his wife, who is a patient. You note the odor of alcohol on his breath and are concerned that the visitor will become violent. You should call for assistance from which of the following departments?
    a. administration
    b. personnel
    c. mechanical services
    d. security

☑ *ANSWERS AND RATIONALE*

10. **(b)** The governing board appoints doctors to the medical staff. p. 18
11. **(b)** The attending physician admits the patient to the hospital. He or she may request a specialist to see and/or treat the patient. pp. 18, 19
12. **(c)** "Resident" is the term used to describe medical school graduates gaining hospital experience. pp. 15, 19
13. **(a)** The case manager coordinates the patient's care from admission to discharge with the insurance company. pp. 14, 22
14. **(b)** An endocrinologist treats glandular diseases. p. 20
15. **(c)** The radiologist, qualified in the use of x-ray and imaging devices, is employed by the diagnostic imaging department. p. 20
16. **(a)** Diagnostic studies related to brain-wave disorders are performed in the neurodiagnostics department. p. 21
17. **(c)** Personnel from the respiratory care department assist in maintaining a patient on a ventilator. p. 22
18. **(b)** The radiation oncology department treats cancerous growths. p. 22
19. **(c)** The health records department, also called the medical records department, is responsible for coding and storing records of discharged patients. p. 22
20. **(b)** The pathology department performs diagnostic procedures on body specimens. p. 22
21. **(d)** Visual examinations of hollow organs or body cavities are performed in the endoscopy department. p. 21
22. **(d)** Call the security department immediately for assistance and notify the nurse in charge. p. 23

23. Which of the following conditions is treated by a gynecologist?
    a. appendicitis
    b. dysmenorrhea
    c. dysentery
    d. nephritis

24. An ophthalmologist treats which of the following conditions?
    a. glaucoma
    b. gastritis
    c. aneurysm
    d. emphysema

25. Disorders of the newborn are treated by a:
    a. neurologist
    b. neonatologist
    c. geriatrist
    d. gastroenterologist

26. Which of the following treats diseases of the aging?
    a. pathologist
    b. osteopath
    c. geriatrist
    d. gastroenterologist

27. Which of the following treats mental illness?
    a. physiatrist
    b. psychiatrist
    c. neurologist
    d. geriatrist

28. A family member of a patient informs you that he has obtained an attorney and is planning to sue the hospital for damages resulting from an incident that involved his father. You should notify which of the following departments?
    a. security
    b. social services
    c. risk management
    d. public relations

29. A "DO" is a:
    a. director of obstetrics
    b. doctor of osteopathy
    c. doctor of orthopedics
    d. director of orthopedics

30. An otolaryngologist specializes in diseases of the:
    a. male reproductive tract
    b. ear, nose, and throat
    c. eye, nose, and throat
    d. esophagus, throat, and stomach

31. Which of the following is an annual requirement of JCAHO for all employees?
    a. TB skin test
    b. updated association membership
    c. flu shot
    d. physical exam

32. The abbreviation PPO means:
    a. post paid officer
    b. prepaid organization
    c. primary provider office
    d. preferred provider organization

33. The abbreviation HMO means:
    a. home maintained operation
    b. health monitor officer
    c. health maintenance organization
    d. home medication order

34. The abbreviation SNF means:
    a. socially nonfunctioning
    b. skilled nursing facility
    c. social nursing faculty
    d. synthetic naturalized foods

☑ *ANSWERS AND RATIONALE*

23. **(b)** A gynecologist treats disorders and diseases of the female reproductive tract. Dysmenorrhea is painful menstruation. p. 20

24 **(a)** An ophthalmologist treats diseases and defects of the eye. Glaucoma is a disease caused by increased pressure within the eye. p. 20

25. **(b)** A neonatologist treats disorders of the newborn. p. 20

26. **(c)** A geriatrist treats diseases of the aging. p. 20

27. **(b)** A psychiatrist diagnoses and treats mental illness. p. 20

28. **(c)** Risk management, which may be part of the quality assurance department, should be notified in such a situation. p. 22

> Risk management, consisting of a variety of proactive efforts to prevent adverse events related to clinical care and facilities operations, is especially focused on avoiding medical malpractice.

29. **(b)** A Doctor of Osteopathy (DO) places special emphasis on the relationship of organs and the musculoskeletal system. p. 18

30. **(b)** An otolaryngologist specializes in diseases of the ear, nose, and throat. p. 20

31. **(a)** A TB skin test is required annually by JCAHO. p. 18

32. **(d)** A PPO, preferred provider organization, is an independent group of physicians or hospitals that provide health care for fees 15% to 20% lower than customary rates. p. 24

33. **(c)** Health maintenance organizations (HMOs) have management responsibility for providing comprehensive health care services on a prepayment basis to voluntarily enrolled persons within a designated population. p. 24

34. **(b)** A skilled nursing facility (SNF) provides care for those patients too sick to go home or to a nursing home but who are not so acutely ill that they require hospitalization. p. 23

TEST-TAKING TIP

> Preparation for the test is vital. Plan for quality study time at a desk or where you feel comfortable. Choose a quiet place, perhaps with your choice of background music. An environment without interruptions is best.

The Nursing Department

1. The person responsible for one or more nursing units for 24 hours a day and whom shift managers report to is called a:
   a. staff nurse
   b. director of nurses
   c. nurse manager
   d. licensed practical nurse

2. You are newly employed and find you need assistance with learning the procedures for your nursing unit. The department that is responsible for orientation and continuing education that may assist you is called:
   a. staff development
   b. nursing service
   c. nursing unit administration
   d. personnel

3. A patient admitted to the hospital with a diagnosis of myocardial infarction would be admitted to the:
   a. DSU
   b. ICU
   c. MICU
   d. CCU

4. You are working on a nursing unit where you transcribe doctors' orders for treatment of cancer. You are working on which of the following units?
   a. drug rehabilitation
   b. psychiatry
   c. oncology
   d. neurology

5. A patient entering the hospital with a head trauma would be admitted to which of the following units?
   a. behavioral health
   b. urology
   c. oncology
   d. neurology

6. A patient entering the hospital with a diagnosis of PID would be admitted to which of the following units?
   a. gynecology
   b. neurology
   c. oncology
   d. urology

7. A patient entering the hospital with a compound fracture of the humerus would be admitted to which of the following units?
   a. medical
   b. oncology
   c. orthopedics
   d. rehabilitation

8. A patient entering the hospital for a TURP would be admitted to which of the following units?
   a. oncology
   b. neurology
   c. gynecology
   d. urology

9. Which of the following nursing personnel carries out the doctor's order to administer an IV medication?
   a. registered nurse
   b. cardiac monitor technician
   c. certified nursing assistant
   d. nurse manager

☑ **ANSWERS AND RATIONALE**

1. **(c)** The nurse manager is the person responsible for one or more nursing units for 24 hours a day.. Other terms for nurse manager are unit manager and clinical manager. pp. 31, 33
2. **(a)** The staff development department, which also may be called the education department, is responsible for continuing education. pp. 32, 33
3. **(d)** The coronary care unit (CCU) cares for patients with heart disease, such as myocardial infarction. p. 34
4. **(c)** Cancer is treated on the oncology unit. p. 34
5. **(d)** A patient with a head trauma would be admitted to the neurology unit. p. 34
6. **(a)** PID is an abbreviation meaning pelvic inflammatory disease; therefore, the patient would be admitted to the gynecology unit. p. 34
7. **(c)** A fracture of the humerus involves the skeletal system; therefore, the patient would be admitted to the orthopedic unit. p. 34
8. **(d)** A transurethral resection of the prostate (TURP) is surgery on the male reproductive tract; therefore, the patient would be admitted to the urology unit. p. 34
9. **(a)** The registered nurse would administer medications, including IV medications. p. 34

10. Which of the following nursing personnel would administer insulin to a patient?
    a. CNA
    b. HUC
    c. RN
    d. PSA

11. The team nursing method of patient care assignment is used on your nursing unit; you would communicate the message that the operating room is ready for Mr. Jones to the:
    a. team member
    b. team leader
    c. attending doctor
    d. nurse manager

12. The primary patient care method of nursing care assignment is used on your nursing unit; you would communicate a patient discharge order to the:
    a. nurse in charge of the unit
    b. nurse caring for the patient
    c. licensed practical nurse
    d. team leader

13. A patient in intensive care is improving and ready to leave the intensive care unit but needs more specialized care than is given on a regular nursing unit. The patient would be transferred to the:
    a. short-stay unit
    b. recovery room
    c. stepdown unit
    d. rehabilitation unit

14. A patient admitted with a diagnosis of Alzheimer's disease would be admitted to:
    a. GYN unit
    b. orthopedics unit
    c. neurology unit
    d. PACU

15. A patient is being admitted with a diagnosis of CVA (stroke). What unit would the patient be assigned to?
    a. orthopedics unit
    b. GYN unit
    c. CCU
    d. neurology unit

16. A patient admitted with an epitheliocarcinoma would be admitted to:
    a. neurology
    b. oncology
    c. orthopedics
    d. rehabilitation

17. A clinical pathway is a/an:
    a. career ladder for nursing
    b. hall leading to the nursing unit
    c. outline of a patient's path for treatment
    d. continuing education for doctors and nurses

18. The term acuity refers to:
    a. a test to determine blood sugar
    b. a disease causing dizziness and loss of hearing
    c. level of care a patient requires
    d. level of hearing

☑ **ANSWERS AND RATIONALE**

10. **(c)** Insulin is a medication; therefore, the RN would administer it. p. 34

> CNA—certified nursing assistant
> PSA—patient support associate
> HUC—health unit coordinator

11. **(b)** The team leader is notified of patient information by the health unit coordinator, and he or she in turn notifies the team members as needed. p. 35
12. **(b)** The nurse caring for the patient is notified. p. 35
13. **(c)** The patient would be transferred to the stepdown unit, where he or she would receive specialized care. p. 34
14. **(c)** Alzheimer's disease is a neurologic disorder; therefore, the patient would be admitted to the neurology unit. p. 34
15. **(d)** A patient with a diagnosis of CVA (cerebral vascular accident) or stroke would be admitted to the neurology unit. p. 34
16. **(b)** Epitheliocarcinoma is a cancerous tumor composed of epithelial cells. The patient would be admitted to oncology. p. 34
17. **(c)** A clinical pathway is an outline of a patient's path for treatment. pp. 31, 36
18. **(c)** Acuity refers to the level of care a patent requires; it is used by nursing for staffing purposes. p. 31

CHAPTER 4

Communication Devices and Their Uses

1. A computer terminal on the nursing unit may be made available for use by:
   a. pressing the "on" button
   b. calling the hospital information systems department
   c. asking the nurse manager to turn it on
   d. entering your identification code and password

2. A list of options projected on the viewing screen of the nursing unit computer is called:
   a. a cursor
   b. a menu
   c. a keyboard
   d. data

3. The flashing symbol on a computer display screen that indicates the position where data may be entered is called the:
   a. password
   b. enter key
   c. cursor
   d. menu

4. Which of the following is the proper way to identify yourself when answering the telephone on the nursing unit?
   a. "4C, may I help you?"
   b. "This is Suzie Smith, 4C."
   c. "Suzie Smith, Health Unit Coordinator, how may I help you?"
   d. "First floor, Suzie Smith, Health Unit Coordinator."

5. When confronted with a question you cannot answer during a telephone conversation, a proper response is:
   a. "May I place you on hold while I get someone to answer that for you?"
   b. "I don't know. Maybe the nurse does."
   c. "I don't know. Do you want me to find out?"
   d. "Hold on a second. Let me see if I can find someone to answer that for you."

6. Which of the following indicates proper telephone etiquette when placing a caller on hold?
   a. "Hang on, please."
   b. "Hold, please."
   c. "I'll place you on hold."
   d. "May I place you on hold?"

7. You have placed the caller on hold. To communicate this to the person who is receiving the call, you should state the:
   a. name of the caller, nature of the call, and incoming line
   b. name and nature of the call only; the incoming line will be flashing
   c. name of the caller and incoming line; the nature of the call can be determined later
   d. incoming line only

☑ ANSWERS AND RATIONALE

1. **(d)** Entering your identification code and password. p. 49
2. **(b)** "Menu" is the name given to a list of options projected on the viewing screen. pp. 44, 49
3. **(c)** The cursor indicates the position where data may be entered. pp. 43, 49
4. **(d)** Stating the nursing unit, your name, and your status is the correct way to identify yourself when answering an incoming call. p. 45
5. **(a)** Asking callers to hold while you find an answer to their question will convey confidence and is good telephone technique. pp. 45, 46
6. **(d)** Asking if you can place the caller on hold is the best customer relations approach. pp. 45, 46
7. **(a)** Giving complete information allows for efficiency and good public relations. p. 46

NOTES

8. When requested by the nurse to place a call to a physician's office, you should plan first by:
   a. recording the patient's name, reason for the call, and name of the person requesting the call
   b. recording the patient's name, reason for the call, physician's office phone number, and name of the nurse requesting the call
   c. recording the patient's name, name of the nurse requesting the call, time, and physician's phone number
   d. advising the nurse to make the call to save confusion

9. Which of the following should *not* be said over the intercom?
   a. "Mr. Butler, your wife called. She will be in to see you at 7:00 tonight."
   b. "Jody, please come to the nurses' station."
   c. "Yes, Mr. Butler, may I help you?"
   d. "Mr. Butler, I need to verify your weight. You are 250 pounds, right?"

10. A telecommunication device that transmits copies of written material over a telephone wire from one site to another is called a:
    a. fax machine
    b. computer
    c. pneumatic tube system
    d. pocket pager

11. You are giving "visiting information" to the father of a patient on your unit. You are the only employee at the nurses' station. The phone rings; you should:
    a. complete the conversation quickly, then answer the phone
    b. excuse yourself from the conversation and answer the phone
    c. let the phone ring; they will call back
    d. continue with the conversation and pick up the phone while finishing the conversation

12. To contact a person by digital pager, you would:
    a. enter a pager number using the computer keyboard and type a message
    b. dial a pager number from a touch-tone phone and dial a number for call back
    c. use the nursing unit intercom and verbally give a pager number for call back
    d. dial a pager number from a touch-tone phone and verbally give a number for call back

13. The health unit coordinator is breaking down a discharged patient's chart to send to the health records department. There are three patient chart forms that do not have any documentation on them. The forms are labeled with the patient's ID label. The health unit coordinator would:
    a. discard them in the unit wastebasket
    b. shred them
    c. leave them with the patient's records and send to health records
    d. cover label with a blank label and leave them in the empty chart to be used for the next patient

14. An example of misuse of e-mail in the workplace would be:
    a. attaching lab results requested by a patient's doctor to his or her office
    b. applying for a position posted on the hospital's Web site
    c. attaching your resume to apply for a teaching position at a university
    d. attaching a work schedule to an e-mail to an instructor who is sending a student down for a clinical rotation.

☑ **ANSWERS AND RATIONALE**

8. **(b)** Having this information at hand allows for the most efficient and effective use of your time. Recording the doctor's office number saves time should the call not be completed because of a busy number, interruptions, and so forth. p. 46

9. **(d)** The patient's weight is confidential in nature. Confidential or sensitive information, such as weight, should not be communicated over the intercom. p. 47

10. **(a)** A fax machine is used to transmit patient information between departments within the hospital and from hospitals to other health care facilities or doctors' offices. p. 48

11. **(b)** Answer the phone as soon as possible by excusing yourself from the conversation. p. 45

12. **(b)** To contact a person by digital pager, dial the pager number from a touch-tone phone. Listen for a ring followed by a series of beeps. Dial your phone number followed by the pound sign (#). pp. 47, 48

> A voice pager is used in the same manner that a digital pager is used, except that, after the series of beeps, a verbal message is given.

13. **(b)** Patient chart forms containing confidential information (patient ID label) that do not have documentation on them must be shredded. p. 48

14. **(c)** Attaching your resume to apply for a teaching position at a university would be considered personal use of the hospital e-mail. p. 51

TEST-TAKING TIP

> The exam is an objective exam, sometimes referred to as a multiple-choice exam. Each question has a stem (the main portion of the question) and four options that either complete the statement or answer the question. There is one correct answer and three possible distracters. The distracters are not meant to trick you, but they may distract you from the correct answer.

Personal and Professional Skills

Communication and Interpersonal Skills

1. A CNA asks you if "423 bed 2" has an order for an oil retention enema. Your best response would be:
   a. "Yes, he does."
   b. "I'll check his chart."
   c. "What is the patient's name?"
   d. "I don't know."

2. An effective technique to use when communicating with someone from a different culture who does not speak English well would be to:
   a. speak louder
   b. use slang, as the person may be more familiar with slang
   c. say nothing and just smile
   d. speak slowly and distinctly

3. A patient on the nursing unit where you are working has been placed in protective isolation. The patient's husband approaches the nursing station and states, "Mary is in isolation! What for? I want to know exactly what is going on here!" Your best response would be:
   a. "Ask her nurse."
   b. "Mary is in isolation for her protection. I will ask her nurse to come in to talk to you."
   c. "I don't know and have nothing to do with patients being placed in isolation."
   d. "Call her doctor and she will explain the reason for the isolation."

4. Which of the following adjectives best describes an assertive person?
   a. opinionated
   b. respectful
   c. forceful
   d. very timid

5. When confronted with an angry telephone caller, your best action would be to:
   a. immediately put the caller on hold and locate the nurse manager to handle it
   b. hang up because it is not your job to deal with such calls
   c. listen to the caller, acknowledge the anger, and document what the caller is saying
   d. hand the phone receiver to the nearest nurse to handle the call

6. What percentage of communication is verbal (actual words used)?
   a. 5%
   b. 10%
   c. 20%
   d. 7%

7. Which of the following best describes what it means to listen with empathy?
   a. to be very patient while the other person is talking
   b. to be sympathetic
   c. to listen and respond with both the heart and mind to understand
   d. to hear only the parts that interest you

☑ ANSWERS AND RATIONALE

1. **(c)** Referring to patients by their room numbers may cause errors in treatment and care and also may interfere with esteem needs. See Maslow's Hierarchy of Needs, p. 60

2. **(d)** Speak slowly and distinctly. p. 65

3. **(b)** Reassure him, and ask Mary's nurse to talk to him—he is concerned that he may contract what Mary has, and he is concerned about her safety. See Maslow's Hierarchy of Needs, p. 59

4. **(b)** An assertive person is respectful of others, the aggressive person is opinionated and forceful, and the nonassertive person is very timid. p. 66–68

5. **(c)** Listen to the caller, acknowledge the anger, and document what is being said. Do not become defensive. If the caller persists, refer him or her to the nurse manager. p. 71

6. **(d)** Only 7% of communication consists of the actual words spoken. p. 61

7. **(c)** Listening with empathy is listening and responding with the heart and mind to truly understand. p. 64

NOTES

8. Which of the following adjectives best describes an aggressive behavior:
   a. respectful
   b. dominating
   c. self-denying
   d. timid

9. A patient stops at the desk to talk and tells you that she is afraid that she has cancer and that her doctor is keeping this information from her. Your best response would be:
   a. tell her not to worry; her doctor is competent
   b. check her chart for any indication that she has cancer, so you can put her mind at ease
   c. tell her she looks well, and everything will be okay
   d. advise her to share her concerns with the doctor, and notify the nurse of her expressed concerns

10. A fellow employee gave a presentation at a staff meeting and afterward shared with you that he felt he did poorly. He gave good information but was obviously nervous and did not present the information well. An appropriate response would be:
    a. "I found your presentation very informative."
    b. "You were pretty nervous."
    c. "I've seen worse."
    d. "Maybe public speaking is not for you."

11. Which of the following is an effective tool to use with an angry telephone caller?
    a. place the caller on hold to allow him or her time to cool down
    b. when answering the phone, identify yourself by nursing unit, name, and status
    c. inform the caller that you are not responsible for everything that happens
    d. tell the caller to calm down and control his or her anger

12. To assume that your race is superior to others is referred to as:
    a. negative assertion
    b. ethnocentrism
    c. stereotyping
    d. fogging

13. You are extremely busy, but a doctor is insistent that you should stop what you are doing to get her a cup of coffee. Your most appropriate response would be:
    a. "I'm not paid to be a waitress."
    b. "Get your own coffee."
    c. "I'll get your coffee in just a minute."
    d. "I'm very busy. The coffee and cups are in the report room. Please help yourself."

14. You notice a visitor smoking in a patient's room where smoking is prohibited. An appropriate way of handling this situation would be for you to say:
    a. "Smoking is not allowed in the hospital. You may go outside if you wish to smoke."
    b. "I'm sorry, but smoking is not allowed— but I won't report it just this once."
    c. "Put out your cigarette. Can't you see the 'no smoking' signs?"
    d. "Put your cigarette out or I'll call security."

15. Dr. Seemore arrives on the nursing unit and loudly announces that his patient, Mr. Polyp, was unable to have his sigmoidoscopy completed because you did not cancel his breakfast tray. Your most appropriate response would be:
    a. "My signature is not the only one on those orders. The nurse should have caught that error."
    b. "I'm so busy and I don't ever get any help around here!"
    c. "I did miss that order. I apologize for the error. Can the sigmoidoscopy be rescheduled for tomorrow?"
    d. "I'm so sorry. I can be so careless and stupid sometimes."

16. Jean, the health unit coordinator who relieves you on a regular basis, has become silent to you, causing an uncomfortable working situation. You would:
    a. ignore the situation and hope that the problem will resolve itself
    b. report the situation to the nurse manager
    c. only speak to Jean when absolutely necessary
    d. ask Jean what the problem is and talk about it

☑ ***ANSWERS AND RATIONALE***

8. **(b)** A person displaying aggressive behavior does not respect others and behaves in a dominating manner. pp. 66–68

9. **(d)** Suggesting the patient share her concerns with her physician is the best response. p. 65

10. **(a)** "I found your presentation very informative" would give constructive feedback. p. 65

11. **(b)** When answering the telephone always identify yourself by nursing unit, name, and status. Doing this puts you on a more personal level with the caller. Also, callers may become even more upset if they need to ask questions to determine whom they are talking to. p. 71

12. **(b)** Ethnocentrism is the inability to accept other cultures—an assumption of cultural superiority. p. 58

13. **(d)** Asking the doctor to help herself is an assertive response. Answers a and b are aggressive, and answer c is nonassertive. pp. 66–68

14. **(a)** Advising the visitors of the rules is the assertive way of handling the situation. Answer b is nonassertive, and answers c and d are both aggressive statements. pp. 66–68

15. **(c)** Admitting the error and offering a solution is the assertive response. Answers a and b are aggressive, and answer d is nonassertive. pp. 66–68

16. **(d)** Ask Jean what the problem is, and talk about it. This is the assertive way of dealing with the situation. pp. 67, 68

NOTES

17. The holiday schedule is posted, and you see that you are scheduled to work more holidays than all the other health unit coordinators on the unit. You would:
    a. say nothing and bring it up on your next evaluation
    b. tell the other health unit coordinators that to be fair they have to give up some of their holidays
    c. do nothing because it's not really important and the other health unit coordinators have children and you don't
    d. go to the staffing office and bring the problem to their attention

18. Pat, a staff nurse with whom you work, is condescending toward you and makes disparaging remarks in conversations about you. You would:
    a. meet with Pat and tell her how you feel about her behavior
    b. refuse to run errands for Pat and ignore her disparaging remarks
    c. report Pat's behavior to the nurse manager
    d. tell Pat you are fed up with her behavior and refuse to talk to her unless absolutely necessary

19. Culturally sensitive care means that:
    a. when a patient is admitted from another country, only nurses from that culture would be assigned to care for that patient
    b. when a patient is from another culture, all health care workers are very aware of what they say and how they say it
    c. all health care workers understand and are sensitive to various cultural differences
    d. when a patient is admitted from a different culture, every effort is made to educate the patient in our culture

20. The most effective way to ensure another that you understand the information that he or she has given to you would be to:
    a. nod your head
    b. smile
    c. paraphrase information
    d. reply with an "OK"

21. A person demonstrating the following type of behavior most of the time probably has a healthy self-esteem:
    a. aggressive
    b. nonassertive
    c. assertive
    d. ethnocentric

22. Which of the following is a behavioral style in which a person stands up for his or her own rights without violating the rights of others:
    a. assertive
    b. aggressive
    c. nonassertive
    d. negative assertion

23. A lady approaches the nurses' station and asks you a question in a different language; your best response would be to:
    a. speak louder because she probably can't understand any English
    b. ask her if she understands any English
    c. tell her that you can't understand what she is saying
    d. tell her that your sorry and that you can't help her

24. To assume that all people who have tattoos or body piercing are gang members is called:
    a. ageism
    b. stereotyping
    c. elitism
    d. negative assertion

25. Using Maslow's Hierarchy of Needs, determine what need this patient is expressing: Patient: "The nurse came in my room last night at 10:00 and took my water away from me. It is 9:00 in the morning and I still haven't had anything to eat or drink!"
    a. self-esteem
    b. physiologic
    c. belonging and love
    d. esteem

ANSWERS AND RATIONALE

17. **(d)** Taking the problem to the staffing office would be the assertive way of solving the problem. It may have been an oversight. pp. 67, 68

18. **(a)** The assertive way of dealing with this problem would be to meet with Pat and express your feelings. pp. 67, 68

19. **(c)** Culturally sensitive care is to understand and be sensitive to others' cultures. pp. 58, 65

20. **(c)** Paraphrasing what you have heard in your own words leaves no doubt that you have understood the sender accurately. p. 64

21. **(c)** An assertive person is confident, respectful of others, and probably has a healthy self-esteem. pp. 67, 68

22. **(a)** An assertive person stands up for their own rights without violating the rights of others. pp. 67, 68

23. **(b)** Ask if she understands English. Do not assume that she can't understand any English. Speaking louder does not help and will cause further confusion and agitation. pp. 65, 66

24. **(b)** Making assumptions based on a person's race, gender, social class, and so on is called stereotyping. p. 58

25. **(b)** The need for food and water is physiologic. p. 58

NOTES

26. Using Maslow's Hierarchy of Needs, determine what need this patient is expressing: Patient: "I've been in the hospital for 3 days and I haven't seen or heard from any of my family since I was admitted."
    a. physiologic
    b. safety and security
    c. esteem
    d. belonging and love

27. Using Maslow's Hierarchy of Needs, determine what need this patient is expressing: Patient: "I don't know if my insurance will pay all of my hospital stay or even if I will have a job when I am well again."
    a. belonging and love
    b. physiologic
    c. safety and security
    d. esteem

28. Using Maslow's Hierarchy of Needs, determine what need this patient is expressing: Patient: "Why don't the nurses take time to listen to me?"
    a. esteem
    b. physiologic
    c. belonging and love
    d. safety and security

29. Someone makes a rude remark to you. Which of the following responses would be considered assertive?
    a. say nothing; it would be best to ignore the remark
    b. "You make me so angry. You always say things that aren't true."
    c. "I probably deserved that."
    d. "I would like to know what you meant by what you said."

30. A nurse comments that you forgot to order the dressing tray that she requested 20 minutes ago. Which of the following responses would be considered nonassertive?
    a. "You expect me to do the work of three people."
    b. "I apologize, I'll do that now."
    c. "I'm sorry I'm so stupid."
    d. "Do it yourself. I'm busy."

31. You are a new employee and the health unit coordinator training you tells you that you are too slow. An assertive response would be:
    a. "I'm new—what do you expect?
    b. "I'm working as fast as I can!"
    c. "I probably do seem slow because I'm not experienced with this computer system yet."
    d. "If you don't want to train me, just say so."

32. According to Maslow's Hierarchy of Needs, a person who feels he or she has reached his or her full potential has met which of the following needs:
    a. physiologic
    b. safety and security
    c. self-actualization
    d. esteem

☑ *ANSWERS AND RATIONALE*

26. **(d)** The patient is expressing belonging and love needs. pp. 59, 60

27. **(c)** The patient is expressing safety and security needs. p. 59

28. **(a)** The patient feels he or she is not being respected and is expressing esteem needs. p. 60

29. **(d)** Asking what the person meant by the rude remark is an assertive response. p. 67

30. **(c)** Putting oneself down is nonassertive. pp. 66, 68

31. **(c)** Admitting that there is some truth to the statement, but not taking it personally, is the assertive response using the fogging skill. p. 70

32. **(c)** A person who feels he or she has reached his or her full potential has reached the self-actualization need. p. 60

NOTES

C
H
A
P
T
E
R

6

Workplace Behavior

Ethics and Legal Concepts

1. One's values are formed by the age of:
   a. 21
   b. 12
   c. 6
   d. 30

2. One of the main purposes of employee performance evaluations is:
   a. to provide feedback with suggestions for improvement
   b. to provide an opportunity for the nurse manager to get acquainted with the employees
   c. to advise employees of all they do wrong
   d. to encourage employees to appreciate their job

3. Which of the following would be most beneficial to you in preparation for your performance evaluation?
   a. be especially efficient when performing your job in the 2 weeks prior to evaluation
   b. treat the nurses and nurse manager especially nice in the 2 weeks prior to evaluation
   c. keep a diary of all accomplishments, classes taken, and in-services attended during the evaluation period
   d. perform additional tasks and work overtime when requested to do so in the 2 weeks prior to evaluation

4. You are the health unit coordinator working on a TICU and you observe a man becoming very agitated and making threatening gestures to one of the nurses. Your immediate response would be to:
   a. walk over to him and ask him to please calm down
   b. call security
   c. ignore him, it's not your concern
   d. walk over and tell the nurse she has a phone call to get her away from the situation

5. Someone makes an inappropriate remark with sexual overtones while touching you on the back. Your best response would be:
   a. slap the person
   b. say nothing and the person will know you aren't interested
   c. report the incident to the nurse manager immediately
   d. tell the person to stop and that you do not welcome his or her behavior

6. You have received a call from a local newspaper reporter, who is inquiring about a celebrity admitted to your unit. You should:
   a. answer the reporter's questions
   b. refer the call to the patient
   c. refer the call to the nurse manager
   d. ask the patient if it is okay to answer the reporter's questions

☑ **ANSWERS AND RATIONALE**

1. **(c)** A person's values are formed by the age of 6. p. 81
2. **(a)** Performance evaluations are mainly to provide feedback and suggestions for improvement. p. 86
3. **(c)** Keep a diary of all accomplishments, classes taken, and in-services attended during the evaluation period. p. 86
4. **(b)** Call security immediately. p. 86

> TICU is an abbreviation for *trauma intensive care unit.*

5. **(d)** The first step is to tell the person to stop and that you do not welcome his or her behavior. p. 86
6. **(c)** Refer the call to the nurse manager. Patient information is protected by the Health Insurance Portability and Accountability Act privacy rule. pp. 83, 84

NOTES

7. A friend of yours has been admitted to the hospital. You know your friend has tested positive for HIV. You should notify:
   a. the friend's doctor
   b. the nurse manager
   c. no one
   d. the nurse caring for the friend

8. A visitor stops by the nursing station and remarks, "My friend Irma seems to be losing a lot of weight. How much does she weigh now?" An appropriate response would be:
   a. "I'm sorry, I can't discuss patient information."
   b. "That is really none of your business."
   c. "Let me look at her chart."
   d. "Why are you asking me? I don't know."

9. Another hospital employee approaches you in the cafeteria to ask the condition and diagnosis of her neighbor, who is a patient on your unit. You should:
   a. tell her to call you at home
   b. tell the employee that you cannot give her that information
   c. since the person is a fellow employee, answer the questions
   d. pretend you don't know the answers

10. The sister of a patient calls the nursing unit and asks what diagnostic procedures have been ordered for her sister. An appropriate response is:
    a. refer the call to her sister's nurse
    b. suggest that she contact her sister's physician
    c. ask her to call later
    d. tell her to ask her sister

11. You receive a call from a man identifying himself as a police officer. He requests a status report on a victim of a gang shooting. The patient has "NINP" written on his chart cover. You should:
    a. refer the call to the nurse manager
    b. hang up immediately
    c. transfer the call to the patient
    d. confirm that the patient is on the unit but you can't give out any information

12. A patient, a victim of spousal abuse, has a restraining order against her husband. You see this man arrive on the nursing unit; your best response would be to:
    a. advise the man to leave the unit immediately
    b. immediately go in to the patient's room and warn her that her husband is coming
    c. do nothing, he could get mad at you
    d. call security immediately

13. You observe a man on the unit that you do not recognize and who is acting strangely. You think he is holding something behind his back; your best reaction would be to:
    a. approach him to ask if you can help him
    b. call an orderly to stand by for protection
    c. notify security immediately
    d. do nothing, it's probably your imagination

14. You notice a professional-looking man who is wearing a suit and tie. You do not recognize him. He is looking at a patient's chart; your best response would be to:
    a. introduce yourself and ask who he is
    b. take the chart from him
    c. tell him that he is not allowed to look at the chart
    d. do nothing; he must be a doctor called in to see the patient

15. A patient comes to the desk and demands to see his chart and states that he knows his rights and that he is entitled to see his chart! Your best response would be to:
    a. advise him that he is not allowed to see his chart
    b. tell him to call his lawyer
    c. advise him that you will notify his nurse and doctor of his request
    d. show him his chart

16. Which of the following statements is helpful in avoiding personal liability while on the job?
    a. have your orders cosigned by the registered nurse
    b. only perform tasks that you have been trained to do and that fall within your job description
    c. always ask the physician to read the orders to you
    d. ask the nurse caring for the patient to verify all orders

☑ *ANSWERS AND RATIONALE*

7. **(c)** You would notify no one; the information is confidential. This information is considered protected health information and is covered by the Health Insurance Portability and Accountability Act privacy rule. pp. 83, 84

8. **(a)** "I'm sorry, I can't discuss patient information." Answering this question would be violating the privacy rule contained in the Health Insurance Portability and Accountability Act. pp. 83, 84

9. **(b)** Tell the employee that you cannot give her that information. Remind her of the confidentiality agreement that you both signed in compliance with the Health Insurance Portability and Accountability Act. pp. 83, 84

10. **(a)** Refer the call to her sister's nurse. Providing patient information would be n violation of the Health Insurance Portability and Accountability Act. pp. 83, 84

11. **(a)** Refer the call to the nurse manager. NINP is an abbreviation for *no information/no publication*. Each patient is given the option of being listed in the hospital directory upon admission to the hospital. pp. 83, 84

12. **(d)** Call security immediately. p. 86

13. **(c)** Call security immediately. p. 86

14. **(a)** Introduce yourself and ask who he is. Protecting the patient's chart is part of the health unit coordinator's responsibility. p. 84

15. **(c)** Advise him that you will notify his nurse and doctor of his request. p. 84

16. **(b)** Only perform tasks that you have been trained to do and that fall within your job description. p. 89

NOTES

17. Which of the following is the legal doctrine that holds the hospital as well as the employee liable for negligence?
    a. *respondeat superior*
    b. standard of care
    c. statute of limitations
    d. tort

18. The person legally responsible for your acts while you are working as a health unit coordinator is:
    a. the charge nurse
    b. the hospital administrator
    c. yourself
    d. the nurse cosigning the orders

19. Which of the following is an example of negligence by a health unit coordinator?
    a. not doing what the nurse requested
    b. transcribing the physician's order incorrectly, resulting in a patient injury
    c. failing to remind the patient's nurse of a previously ordered daily treatment
    d. taking longer breaks than he or she was entitled to

20. An informed consent means that the:
    a. surgery department has been informed and the procedure is scheduled
    b. surgery procedure to be done has been written as an order by the physician
    c. person signing the consent has been informed of the risks and characteristics of the procedure and understands them
    d. nurse responsible for obtaining the appropriate signature has been informed

21. Which of the following is involved when a situation occurs that is in conflict with your personal value system?
    a. ethics
    b. legalities
    c. negligence
    d. tort

22. There is a physician whose writing is very difficult to read and who writes orders for patients on the unit where you work. You should:
    a. ask the physician to print his orders
    b. report the physician to the medical board
    c. ask the physician to please wait while you read his orders prior to his leaving the nursing unit
    d. depend on the nurses to assist you in interpreting the orders

23. The nursing unit is understaffed. A nurse asked you to help her out by taking a medication in to a patient. You should:
    a. ask the patient if he or she would mind taking the medication from you even if you are not licensed
    b. take the medication to the patient as a favor to the nurse
    c. advise the nurse that you are not licensed to administer medication
    d. check if other health unit coordinators in the hospital take medications to patients

24. Accountability can be defined as:
    a. being answerable for what you have done
    b. values, rules of conduct
    c. a law
    d. professional negligence

25. You have been informed by risk management that you are to give a pretrial statement as a witness to an incident that occurred on your unit. This is called a/an:
    a. testament
    b. deposition
    c. tort
    d. informed consent

☑ **ANSWERS AND RATIONALE**

17. **(a)** *Respondeat superior,* which means "let the master respond," holds the hospital as well as the employee liable for negligence. p. 80

18. **(c)** You are legally responsible for your acts while working as a health unit coordinator. p. 89

19. **(b)** Incorrectly transcribing a physician's order is an example of negligence. p. 89

20. **(c)** The person signing the consent has been informed of the risks and characteristics of the procedure and understands them. Informed consent is a mandatory prerequisite for any invasive procedure or surgery. pp. 80, 89

21. **(a)** An ethical dilemma is a situation that presents a conflicting moral claim. p. 88

22. **(c)** Ask the physician to please wait while you read his orders prior to his leaving the nursing unit. p. 89

23. **(c)** Only a licensed health care provider may administer medication. p. 89

24. **(a)** Accountability is being answerable to someone for something you have done. p. 80

25. **(b)** A deposition is a pretrial statement given by a witness under oath. p. 80

TEST-TAKING TIP

Read the stem of the question, and then read each option as if it were a separate true-false statement. Eliminate the options you know to be false and choose the best of the remaining answers. Look for choices that give complete information.

Management Techniques and Problem-Solving Skills for Health Unit Coordinating

1. You have just arrived on the nursing unit. Which of the following tasks that need to be done should you do first?
   a. relay the message to the nurse that surgery is sending for his or her patient
   b. order a stat CBC
   c. obtain a lab result for the doctor
   d. transcribe a discharge order

2. You return to the nursing unit from a break to find several new written orders. Which order would you start with?
   a. CMP and CBC this AM
   b. discharge order
   c. reg diet
   d. PA & Lat chest x-ray today

3. How can you best keep track of the whereabouts of a patient's chart?
   a. make a notation on the census worksheet
   b. rely on your memory
   c. depend on each nurse to keep track of his or her patients' charts
   d. it is not your responsibility to track patient charts

4. You would use a note pad to:
   a. list the tasks you are unable to complete momentarily
   b. assist you to remember difficult procedures
   c. record difficult-to-remember phone and pager numbers
   d. list routine phone numbers

5. An angry visitor approaches the nursing station and complains to you that her mother has not had a bath for 2 days. The appropriate response is:
   a. refer the visitor to her mother's nurse immediately; no need to waste your time listening
   b. listen to the complaint, then explain that patient care is not your responsibility
   c. advise the visitor to report the incident to her mother's physician; he or she will take care of it
   d. listen to the visitor, tell her you understand her complaint, and then ask her to wait while you get her mother's nurse

6. Which of the following would you record on the census worksheet?
   a. lab results
   b. DNR
   c. physician's name
   d. patient diagnosis

7. You find that the nursing station could be more functional if the chart forms were located closer to the charts. You should:
   a. discuss the change with the nurse manager
   b. move the chart forms and listen for feedback
   c. take a poll to see if everyone is in agreement
   d. leave the chart forms where they are; they were placed there for a reason

☑ ANSWERS AND RATIONALE

1. **(a)** Relay the message to the nurse that surgery is sending for his or her patient. pp. 102, 103
2. **(b)** Transcribe the discharge order first so that the clerical work can be processed. pp. 102, 103
3. **(a)** Record the time the patient's chart leaves the unit and its destination on the census worksheet beside the patient's name. p. 100
4. **(a)** Tasks you are unable to complete momentarily should be recorded on the note pad. p. 104
5. **(d)** Respond to the visitor's initial remarks by listening and showing that you care, and then refer her to the appropriate person for further assistance. pp. 100–102
6. **(b)** DNR (do not resuscitate) is information you may use during the shift. p. 100
7. **(a)** Discuss your idea with the nurse manager first. p. 105

NOTES

8. You arrive on the nursing unit to find several charts out of the rack lying around the nursing unit. Which of the following should you do *first*?
   a. replace all charts in the rack except the charts that are flagged
   b. check each chart for new orders flagged or not
   c. leave the charts as you found them until you have a lot of time to look at them
   d. take one chart at a time and transcribe all new orders, and return the chart to the rack when completed

9. Nursing unit personnel should record nursing unit items that are running low on the:
   a. supply needs list
   b. patient activity sheet
   c. memory sheet
   d. census

10. A visitor approaches the nurses' station and asks you if his father may have a piece of chocolate candy. You should first:
    a. refer the visitor to his father's nurse
    b. say "Yes, it's just one piece of candy"
    c. check the father's diet on the patient's Kardex form or in the computer
    d. ask the father if he has been eating candy

11. You observe a visitor entering an isolation patient's room without following proper procedure. You should:
    a. call the patient's nurse
    b. advise the visitor of the proper procedure
    c. ignore the situation since it is not your responsibility
    d. tell the visitor to read the signs

12. A very hostile visitor approaches the nursing station with the complaint that her daughter has been ignored and treated rudely by the CNA. You should:
    a. reprimand the CNA
    b. explain to the visitor that the CNA is overworked and that she didn't mean to be rude
    c. advise the visitor to take the complaint to her daughter's physician
    d. listen to the visitor's complaint, tell her you understand how she feels, and then get the appropriate team leader

13. You find the unit is getting very busy and you are out of admission charts. An appropriate action would be:
    a. skip your lunch break and assemble more admission charts
    b. call another unit for help
    c. call the nurse manager for help
    d. ask a volunteer to assemble more admission charts

14. The mother of a terminally ill child relates to you that she and her family are very upset about the level of noise and apparent "partying" that was taking place on the critical care unit the day before. An appropriate response would be:
    a. "The staff are really burned out and need to let loose now and then."
    b. "They do get carried away; I'm sorry that they were so inconsiderate."
    c. "I understand what you are telling me and I will ask the nurse manager to come in and talk to you."
    d. "I wasn't here yesterday."

15. Which of the following tasks would take priority over the others?
    a. a stat CBC
    b. pre-op orders
    c. calling a code arrest for a patient when requested to do so
    d. a discharge order

16. Ergonomics is a term meaning:
    a. the study of work to make the workplace more comfortable and to improve health and productivity
    b. the assessment of medical care costs
    c. a diagnostic hearing examination to determine hearing loss
    d. a physical therapy examination to measure a patient's flexibility

17. A central service credit slip is:
    a. a reward for employees for outstanding performance
    b. a form to obtain additional supplies from the central service department
    c. a form used to credit a patient's account for unused items that were previously charged to him or her
    d. a form used to add an additional charge to a patient's account

☑ **ANSWERS AND RATIONALE**

8. **(b)** Always check all charts out of the rack for new orders. Busy doctors can easily forget to flag charts with new orders. p. 103

9. **(a)** Needed items are to be recorded on a supply needs list (list may be computerized). p. 98

10. **(c)** Check the father's diet order on the Kardex form or in the computer. If there is any doubt, ask the patient's nurse. p. 101

11. **(b)** It is the responsibility of the health unit coordinator to communicate patient information to visitors. pp. 100–102

12. **(d)** Listening and responding appropriately is the first step in handling a visitor's complaint. p. 100–102

13. **(d)** Ask a volunteer (if available) to assemble more admission charts. p. 106

14. **(c)** It is important to present a caring attitude and not become defensive. Your initial handling of a customer complaint often determines how far the complaint will go. pp. 100–102

15. **(c)** A patient in crisis takes priority over all other tasks. p. 103

16. **(a)** Ergonomics is the study of work to make the workplace more comfortable and to improve health and productivity. pp. 96, 104

17. **(c)** a central service credit slip is a form used to credit a patient's account for unused items that were previously charged to him or her. pp. 96, 98

NOTES

18. A nursing unit census sheet is a:
    a. list of patient names, including their ages and the names of their doctors
    b. list of doctors on hospital staff that may admit patients to the nursing unit
    c. list of nursing staff employed at hospital that may work on the nursing unit
    d. list of patient names, including their age and their diagnoses

19. Reusable equipment that is discontinued would be stored in the:
    a. patient's room until picked up by a central service technician
    b. nursing unit hallway until picked up by a central service technician
    c. dirty utility room until picked up by a central service technician
    d. nurse's station until picked up by a central service technician

20. The health unit coordinator's responsibility regarding the crash or code cart may be to:
    a. check dates on medications
    b. test emergency equipment to make sure all is in working order
    c. take inventory of what is on the cart
    d. order supplies and/or medication as requested by the nurse

21. Which of the following techniques would be helpful to prevent cumulative injuries?
    a. take longer breaks
    b. work standing up half the time
    c. take frequent mini-breaks
    d. bring a pillow to sit on while working

22. Brainstorming is a method used by a group to:
    a. evaluate who is the smartest employee
    b. identify new ideas
    c. argue in a structured way
    d. share gossip

23. An effective time management technique is to:
    a. plan for rush periods
    b. skip your breaks
    c. try to do several tasks at the same time
    d. leave routine tasks for the next shift

24. A stress-management technique that would assist you on the job is:
    a. tell nurses and doctors that you are too busy to help them
    b. speak your mind; tell people to please leave you alone
    c. take extra breaks
    d. ask for help when you need it

☑ *ANSWERS AND RATIONALE*

18. **(a)** the nursing unit census would include a list of patient names, their age, and the names of their doctors. The patients' diagnoses would not be listed on the nursing unit census. p. 96

19. **(c)** discontinued equipment would be stored in the dirty utility room until picked up by a central service technician. p. 97

20. **(d)** order supplies and/or medication as requested by the nurse. pp. 99, 100

21. **(c)** take frequent mini-breaks, stand, walk, and stretch your back and legs at least every hour. These small breaks in position help avoid neuromuscular strain and alleviate the tension of job stress. pp. 104, 105

22. **(b)** brainstorming is a structured group activity that allows three to ten people to tap into the creativity of the group to identify new ideas. Typically in quality improvement, the technique is used to identify probable causes and possible solutions of quality problems. p. 96

23. **(a)** take time at the beginning of each day to plan for anticipated rush periods. Examples of rush periods would be in the morning while the doctors are making rounds and in the afternoon when new admissions arrive. pp. 105, 106

24. **(d)** ask for help when you need it. p. 106

NOTES

The Patient's Chart and Transcription of Doctors' Orders

The Patient's Chart

1. Which of the following is a standard patient chart form and is included in an admission packet?
   a. consent form
   b. anticoagulant record
   c. physician's order sheet
   d. diabetic record

2. Which of the following is a supplemental patient chart form that should only be used if needed?
   a. physician's order sheet
   b. physician's progress record
   c. history and physical (H&P) sheet
   d. parenteral fluid or infusion record

3. Upon discharge, the patient's chart is sent to the:
   a. business office to determine charges
   b. physician's office to be available for follow-up care
   c. health records department to be stored
   d. home care department to be stored and/or used for home care

4. An inpatient is a patient who:
   a. is admitted to a hospital for 12 hours or more
   b. is admitted to a hospital for 24 hours or more
   c. is admitted to a hospital for any length of time
   d. receives health care from the hospital

5. A discharged patient's labeled chart form that does not have any documentation on it should be:
   a. sent to health records with the rest of the chart
   b. thrown in the wastebasket
   c. shredded
   d. relabeled and used for another patient

6. Twelve midnight in military time is:
   a. 1200
   b. 0120
   c. 0024
   d. 2400

7. Three-thirty in the afternoon in military time is:
   a. 0330
   b. 1630
   c. 1530
   d. 3300

8. A patient receiving heparin would require which of the following forms placed on his or her chart?
   a. diabetic record
   b. clinical pathway record
   c. anticoagulant therapy record
   d. respiratory care therapy record

☑ *ANSWERS AND RATIONALE*

1. **(c)** Standard patient chart forms are those commonly used on all patients' charts. A physician's order sheet is used to indicate care and treatment for a hospitalized patient. pp. 122, 126

2. **(d)** Supplemental patient chart forms are used depending on the patient's care and treatment. The parenteral fluid or infusion record is considered a supplemental form. pp. 146, 148

3. **(c)** The discharged patient's chart is sent to the health records department, where it is indexed and stored. p. 119

4. **(b)** An inpatient is a patient who is admitted for 24 hours or more. p. 118

5. **(c)** Any discarded patient chart form labeled with patient information must be shredded to protect patient confidentiality. p. 152

6. **(d)** 2400 is 12:00 midnight in military time. p. 119

7. **(c)** 1530 is 3:30 PM in military time. p. 119

8. **(c)** Heparin is an anticoagulant, so an anticoagulant therapy record would be required. pp. 142, 144

NOTES

9. A patient's physician's order sheet with written orders on it has been labeled with the wrong patient ID label. You should:
   a. discard the order sheet and ask the physician to rewrite the orders
   b. draw an X across the incorrect label; write date, time, "mistaken entry," first initial, last name; and place the correct label next to or under the incorrect label
   c. place the correct label over the incorrect label
   d. rewrite the orders and ask the nurse to sign them with the doctor's name

10. A patient receiving an intravenous infusion will have which of the following forms placed on his or her chart?
    a. therapy record
    b. anticoagulant therapy record
    c. diabetic record
    d. parenteral fluid record

11. Which of the following is the correct recording on a surgical consent form?
    a. lt hip arthroplasty
    b. lt hip arthoplasty
    c. left hip arthroplasty
    d. left hip arthoplasty

12. Which of the following is the health unit coordinator's responsibility for maintaining the patient's chart?
    a. keep the chart where it can be seen at all times
    b. know the identity of persons having access to the charts
    c. document nursing treatments on the nursing progress notes
    d. document patient complaints on the nursing progress notes

13. Which of the following forms is signed by the patient on admission to serve as a financial agreement and would set forth the general services that the hospital will provide?
    a. face sheet
    b. conditions of admission
    c. advance directive
    d. DRG sheet

14. A red tape placed on a patient's chart with "name alert" written on it would indicate:
    a. the patient's last name has been misspelled
    b. the patient's last name is extremely difficult to spell
    c. there is more than one patient on the unit with the same or similarly spelled last name
    d. the patient has used aliases

15. An "old record" refers to a:
    a. record of a patient who is over 50 years old
    b. record of a patient from more than 7 years ago
    c. patient's record from a previous admission
    d. record of a patient's hospital stay from the first day of admission

16. A Walla Roo is a:
    a. locked patient chart rack located outside the patient's door
    b. chart rack located at the nurses' station
    c. chart rack located in the patient's room
    d. portable chart holder

17. The term "stuffing" a patient's chart indicates that the health unit coordinator will:
    a. place additional blank patient chart forms in the chart
    b. take forms out of the patient's chart that are no longer needed
    c. place the chart in the patient chart rack
    d. place patient ID labels on all the patient chart forms in the chart

18. The term "clinical pathway" refers to:
    a. the distance from admitting to the nursing unit a patient is admitted to
    b. the name of the hospital newsletter
    c. a computer menu of order options
    d. a form that includes the physician's orders, a plan of care with treatment, and predicted outcomes

19. Which of the following forms provides patient information, including insurance information, patient home address, and home telephone numbers of nearest of kin?
    a. face sheet
    b. conditions of admissions form
    c. advance directive checklist
    d. nurse's admission notes

☑ ANSWERS AND RATIONALE

9. **(b)** Draw an X through the incorrect patient ID label; write date, time, "mistaken entry," first initial, and last name; and place the correct label next to or under the incorrect label. p. 152

> Chart forms (with notations on them) that have been labeled with an incorrect patient ID label card may not be removed. The correct label may be placed next to or below the incorrect label. It is also permissible to print the information in ink by hand. After the correct label or information has been placed on the chart form, an X should be made across the incorrect information and "mistaken entry" written above the first line. The date, time, your first initial, your last name, and your status should appear next to the words "mistaken entry."

10. **(d)** The parenteral fluid sheet, or infusion record, is used by the nurse to record the types and amounts of intravenous fluid administered to the patient. pp. 146, 148

11. **(c)** Left hip arthroplasty is not abbreviated and is the correctly spelled procedure for a surgical consent form. pp. 146, 148

12. **(b)** It is the health unit coordinator's responsibility to know the identity of persons having access to the patient's chart. p. 120

13. **(b)** The conditions of admission (COA or C of A) would be signed on admission. p. 122

14. **(c)** A piece of red tape with "name alert" indicates that there is more than one patient on the unit with the same last name and extra attention should be paid by caregivers not to confuse the charts. p. 118

15. **(c)** An "old record" refers to the patient's record from a previous admission. p. 118

16. **(a)** A Walla Roo is a locked chart rack located on the wall outside of a patient's room which stores the patient's chart and when unlocked forms a shelf to write upon. pp. 118, 121

17. **(a)** "Stuffing" a chart indicates that the HUC will place additional blank patient forms on the patient's chart for use when needed. pp. 118, 155

18. **(d)** The clinical pathway is a form that includes the physician's orders, a plan of care with treatment, and predicted outcomes. Clinical pathways are preestablished based on the patient's medical diagnosis. pp. 142, 143

19. **(a)** The face sheet provides patient information, including insurance information, patient home address, and home telephone numbers of nearest of kin. pp. 121, 122

20. Taking older forms out of a patient's chart to make it more manageable is a process called:
    a. stuffing the chart
    b. thinning the chart
    c. editing the chart
    d. monitoring the chart

21. Which of the following forms records the patient's past illnesses, surgeries, and symptomatic history?
    a. face sheet
    b. history and physical (H&P)
    c. conditions of admission
    d. medication administration record

22. The patient's height, weight, and allergies will be found on which of the following forms?
    a. nurse's admission form
    b. face sheet
    c. admission and agreement form
    d. patient ID bracelet

23. To thin a patient's chart you would follow the procedure as outlined in:
    a. your job description
    b. the policy and procedure manual
    c. the nursing unit communication book
    d. the employee handbook

24. Forms removed when "thinning" a patient's chart would be:
    a. discarded
    b. shredded
    c. sent immediately to the health records department
    d. placed in a properly labeled envelope and stored on the nursing unit until the patient is transferred or discharged

☑ *ANSWERS AND RATIONALE*

20. **(b)** Thinning a chart is the process of taking older forms out of a patient's chart to make it more manageable. pp. 118, 155

21. **(b)** The patient's H&P (history and physical) would have a record of the patient's past illnesses, surgeries, and present symptomatic history. pp. 130, 140

22. **(a)** The nurse's admission form would have the patient's admission height, weight, and allergies recorded. pp. 127, 128

23. **(b)** Procedures are outlined in the policy and procedure manual. p. 155

24. **(d)** The removed forms would be placed in an envelope labeled with the patient's ID label and dated, notated for time, and initialed by the health unit coordinator who thinned the chart. The removed forms would be kept on the unit until the patient is discharged and then would be sent to health records with the rest of the patient's chart. p. 155

NOTES

Transcription of Doctors' Orders

1. A new set of doctor's orders can be recognized by the chart being:
   a. open
   b. in the rack
   c. flagged
   d. out of the rack

2. Which of the following is a "standing order"?
   a. Demerol 50 mg IM q 4h prn for severe pain
   b. Avalide 300 mg/12.5 mg, 1 PO qd
   c. NPO 2400 hrs
   d. CXR PA and LAT in AM

3. Which of the following is a "standing prn order"?
   a. Phenergan 25 mg IM q 4h for N/V
   b. CMP in AM
   c. Cefadyl 1 g IV q 6h
   d. Ambien 5 mg PO at hs tonight

4. "Lomotil tab 1 PO qid until diarrhea subsides" is which of the following?
   a. a standing order
   b. a prn order
   c. a one-time or short-order series
   d. a stat order

5. The purpose of the Kardex form is to:
   a. document patient progress
   b. maintain a current profile of patient information
   c. order patient supplies and treatments
   d. document patient medications

6. Symbols are used in the transcription procedure to:
   a. indicate completion of each transcription step
   b. notify the doctor that the orders are transcribed
   c. notify the nurse that the orders are transcribed
   d. allow the nurse to evaluate the health unit coordinator

7. The process of recording data on the doctor's order sheet to indicate completion of transcription is called:
   a. flagging
   b. kardexing
   c. requisitioning
   d. signing-off

8. Symbols are recorded on the doctor's order sheet:
   a. after the transcription of all the orders
   b. before beginning each transcription step
   c. after finishing each transcription step
   d. after the RN signs-off the orders

9. When in doubt about the interpretation of a doctor's order, you should:
   a. check with the patient to find out what the doctor told him or her
   b. avoid calling the doctor if possible, since this wastes his or her time and yours
   c. check with the patient's nurse or doctor
   d. go with what you think, especially if it is not a critical type of order

☑ **ANSWERS AND RATIONALE**

1. **(c)** "Flagging" is the term used to describe the practice of identifying a patient's chart that has new doctor's orders recorded on the doctor's order sheet. p. XXX Sometimes physicians or residents forget to flag new orders. It is good practice for the health unit coordinator to check every chart for new orders prior to returning it to the rack. pp. 160, 161

2. **(b)** Avalide 300 mg/12.5 mg , 1 PO qd is a standing order that will be in effect until a discontinue or change order is written by the doctor. pp. 161, 163

3. **(a)** The qualifying phrase "for N/V" (nausea and vomiting) makes this a prn order, which will be executed according to the patient's needs. p. 163

4. **(c)** The qualifying phase "until diarrhea subsides" would make this a one-time or short-order series (if the order read "for diarrhea," the order would be prn). p. 163

5. **(b)** The purpose of the Kardex form is to maintain a current profile of patient information (some hospitals are using computerized kardexing). p. 160, 163–165

6. **(a)** Symbols are used to indicate completion of each transcription step. Since transcription, especially of a long set of doctor's orders, involves many steps, and since the health unit coordinator is often interrupted, using symbols assists in avoiding errors of omission. pp. 161, 166

7. **(d)** Signing-off indicates completion of transcription of a set of doctor's orders. pp. 160, 166, 167

8. **(c)** Symbols are recorded after completion of each step of transcription. If not done at this time, the usefulness of symbols is negated. p. 166

9. **(c)** When in doubt about a doctor's order, always check with the doctor or the patient's nurse. p. 172

NOTES

10. Which of the following is a reasonable method to rely on to assure that you do not miss any written orders during the transcription process?
    a. always insist that doctors and/or residents read their orders to you prior to leaving the unit
    b. ask the patient's nurse to verify that your interpretation of the orders is correct
    c. when orders are written on the top of the physician's order sheet, check the previous order sheet to make sure they are not continued
    d. ask another health unit coordinator to read orders with you

11. In the doctor's order "Lytes now," it would be ordered:
    a. as soon as possible
    b. with the patient's next routine blood draw
    c. at the nurse's earliest convenience
    d. stat

12. You arrive on the nursing unit and find that several doctors have made rounds on their patients and have written orders on several charts. You would:
    a. take one chart at a time and transcribe all the orders
    b. read all the orders, send copies or fax orders to the pharmacy as necessary, order stats, and then take one chart at a time and transcribe the rest of the orders
    c. read all the orders, order all tests that need to be ordered, and then transcribe the rest of the orders one chart at a time
    d. call the nurse manager and ask for help

☑ **ANSWERS AND RATIONALE**

10. **(c)** Orders can easily be missed when written on the bottom of a doctor's order sheet and continued on the next page. p. 172

11. **(d)** "Now" orders are usually considered the same as stat orders and should receive urgent attention. p. 163

12. **(b)** Read the complete set of doctor's orders for all doctors. Send the pharmacy copies or fax the doctors' orders as necessary, order stats, and then proceed to transcribe all other orders that will ensure that patients will receive their medications on time and that stat orders will be done as ordered. p. 170

NOTES

CHAPTER 10

Patient Activity, Patient Positioning, and Nursing Observation Orders

1. A pulse obtained at the wrist is called a/an:
   a. radial pulse
   b. pulse rate
   c. apical pulse
   d. pedal pulse

2. I & O is the measurement of the patient's:
   a. food intake and output
   b. fluid intake and fluid output
   c. intravenous intake and urine output
   d. oral intake and urine output

3. Which of the following is a patient activity order?
   a. log roll
   b. wt daily
   c. NVS q 2h
   d. OOB

4. Which of the following is the abbreviation for "every other day"?
   a. qd
   b. qod
   c. qid
   d. q 24h

5. Which of the following is the abbreviation for "as desired"?
   a. as de
   b. ad lib
   c. as tol
   d. prn

6. "VS q 4h" means taking:
   a. temperature, pulse, respiration, and blood pressure four times a day
   b. temperature, pulse, and respiration four times a day
   c. temperature, pulse, and respiration every 4 hours
   d. temperature, pulse, respiration, and blood pressure every 4 hours

7. Which of the following indicates the patient is not to be out of bed?
   a. BRP
   b. CBR
   c. CBC
   d. OOB

8. Which of the following means "two times a day"?
   a. qid
   b. tid
   c. bid
   d. qd

9. Which of the following would be an appropriate nursing observation order for a patient admitted with a contusion or head trauma?
   a. CVP
   b. PCA
   c. NVS
   d. PAS

☑ *ANSWERS AND RATIONALE*

1. **(a)** The radial pulse is obtained at the wrist. p. 177
2. **(b)** Intake and output (I & O) is the measurement of the patient's total fluid intake, whether oral or intravenous, and the patient's fluid output, including urine, emesis, wound drainage, and other types of fluid output. pp. 177, 183
3. **(d)** "OOB," or out of bed, is a patient activity order. p. 178
4. **(b)** "qod" is the abbreviation for every other day. p. 178
5. **(b)** "ad lib" is the abbreviation for "as desired." p. 178
6. **(d)** "VS q 4h" means taking temperature, pulse, respiration, and blood pressure every 4 hours. p. 178
7. **(b)** "CBR" is the abbreviation for complete bed rest; therefore, the patient is not to be out of bed. p. 178
8. **(c)** "bid" means two times a day. p. 178
9. **(c)** Neurologic vital signs (NVS), the measurement of the function of the body's neurologic system, include checking pupils of the eye, verbal response, and so forth, and would be appropriate for a patient admitted with a contusion or head trauma (CVP—central venous pressure; PCA—patient-controlled analgesia; PAS—pulsatile antiembolism stockings). pp. 177, 178

NOTES

10. A pulse oximeter is used to measure a patient's:
    a. oxygen saturation of arterial blood
    b. temperature
    c. pulse rate
    d. blood pressure

11. When a patient is determined to be "febrile," he or she:
    a. has a fever
    b. does not have a fever
    c. does not have control of body functions
    d. does have control of body functions

12. An aural temperature is one taken:
    a. rectally
    b. orally
    c. under the arm
    d. in the ear

13. A notation that the patient is A & O would indicate that the patient is:
    a. awake and outspoken
    b. alert and oriented
    c. attended to and outpatient
    d. attentive and open

14. The apical pulse rate is defined as the:
    a. pulse rate taken at the wrist
    b. heart sounds heard at the midline of the chest
    c. pulse rate felt at the top of the foot
    d. pulse rate heard at the heart's apex

15. A bedside commode is a/an:
    a. type of wheelchair
    b. special chair for paralyzed patients
    c. open-seated bedside chair for toilet use
    d. special chair for bathing the patient

16. An observation of a patient's verbal responses and checking eye pupils is referred to as:
    a. cardinal vascular signs
    b. neurologic vital signs
    c. routine vital signs
    d. respiratory symptoms

17. The pulse rate taken on the top of the foot is called the:
    a. radial pulse
    b. carotid pulse
    c. femoral pulse
    d. pedal pulse

☑ *ANSWERS AND RATIONALE*

10. **(a)** A pulse oximeter measures the oxygen saturation of arterial blood. pp. 177, 184

11. **(a)** Febrile would indicate that the patient has an elevated temperature or a fever. Afebrile would indicate no fever. p. 177

12. **(d)** An aural temperature would be taken in the ear (tympanic membrane temperature). p. 183

13. **(b)** "A & O" is an abbreviation meaning alert and oriented. p. 178

14. **(d)** The apical pulse is taken at the heart's apex. p. 177

15. **(c)** A bedside commode (BSC) is an open-seated bedside chair for toilet use. pp. 177, 178

16. **(b)** Neurologic vital signs (NVS) include the observation of a patient's verbal responses and checking eye pupils. p. 178

17. **(d)** The pedal pulse rate is taken at the top of the foot. pp. 177, 184

NOTES

Nursing Treatment Orders

1. The hospital department responsible for the distribution of supplies used for nursing procedures is:
   a. purchasing
   b. mechanical services
   c. business office
   d. central service

2. Reusable equipment should be promptly returned to the central service department to avoid:
   a. excessive patient charges
   b. contaminating other patients
   c. clutter in the utility room
   d. inaccurate inventory

3. When the nurse executes the order "TWE HS," he or she will:
   a. insert a tube into the patient's urethra
   b. restrain the patient
   c. introduce fluid into the patient's rectum
   d. give the patient a bedtime snack

4. Colostomy irrigation is used to:
   a. remove stomach contents
   b. relieve gastric pressure
   c. wash out the urinary bladder
   d. regulate the discharge of stool

5. An indwelling or Foley catheter may also be referred to as what type of catheter?
   a. retention
   b. Hoffman
   c. nonretention
   d. residual

6. The order "cath for residual" requires the nurse to catheterize the patient:
   a. upon rising
   b. after voiding
   c. to determine patency
   d. after bladder irrigation

7. A Harris flush is a/an:
   a. type of portable toilet
   b. device used for wound irrigations
   c. ear irrigation
   d. return-flow enema used to relieve distention

8. The doctor's order states the IV is to run at 100 cc/hr. You need to order the IV solution for the next 24 hours. How many 1000-cc bags would you order?
   a. one
   b. two
   c. three
   d. four

9. D_5LR means:
   a. 5% distilled water with lactated Ringer's
   b. 5% dextral with lactated Ringer's
   c. 5% dioxin with lactated Ringer's
   d. 5% dextrose with lactated Ringer's

10. The doctor ordered an IV of 1000 cc of D_5W @ 125 cc/hr. How many hours would it take to infuse?
    a. 8
    b. 10
    c. 12
    d. 14

☑ ANSWERS AND RATIONALE

1. **(d)** The central service department (CSD) distributes the supplies used for nursing procedures (may also be referred to as SPD, or supply purchasing department). p. 191

2. **(a)** Patients are usually charged a rental fee for reusable equipment; therefore, promptly returning the equipment to central service after it is discontinued will avoid extra charges to the patient. p. 192

3. **(c)** TWE is the abbreviation for tap-water enema. An enema is the introduction of fluid into the rectum. p. 190

4. **(d)** A colostomy is an artificial opening into the colon that allows for the passage of stool. It acts as a substitute for the rectum and anus. Usually the rectum has been surgically removed. Colostomy irrigation regulates the discharge of stool through the colostomy. p. 194

5. **(a)** A Foley catheter is a type of indwelling or retention catheter. The catheter remains in the bladder and is usually connected to a continuous drainage system. pp. 189, 195

6. **(b)** Residual is the amount of urine remaining in the bladder after voiding; therefore, the patient is catheterized immediately after voiding to determine the amount of urine, if any, remaining in the bladder. p. 195

7. **(d)** A Harris flush is a return-flow enema used to relieve distention. p. 193

8. **(c)** To determine the number of bags needed, divide the amount in the bag by the number of cc's to be administered per hour: 1000 cc, 100 cc/hr = 10 hr. To cover 24 hours, three bags are needed. p. 199

9. **(d)** D_5LR means 5% dextrose with lactated Ringer's. p. 189

10. **(a)** For the answer, divide 1000 by 125. The correct answer is 8 hr. p. 199

NOTES

11. The doctor's order reads 1000 cc of LR @ 125 cc/hr × 3 days. How many 1000-cc bags would need to be ordered to cover the 3 days?
    a. 9
    b. 10
    c. 11
    d. 12

12. Which of the following solutions is most commonly used along with administering blood?
    a. D_5LR
    b. D/W
    c. 0.45 NS
    d. LR

13. It is 2:00 PM. You have just returned to your unit from picking up blood from the blood bank. The nurse states that, because of an emergency on the unit, the blood will not be started during the shift that ends at 3:30 PM. You would:
    a. leave the blood on the desk with the requisition
    b. return the blood to the blood bank
    c. put the blood in the unit refrigerator
    d. place the blood with the patient's IV solutions

14. Which of the following is *not* a transfusion order?
    a. fresh frozen plasma
    b. cryoprecipitates
    c. LE cell prep
    d. plasma

15. Another name for an intermittent IV line is a:
    a. Heplock
    b. J-P
    c. Hemovac
    d. venipuncture

16. NG tube used for suctioning purposes would be connected to a/an:
    a. IV infusion pump
    b. kangaroo pump
    c. wall suction
    d. Pleur-evac

17. To transcribe the order "keep Hemovac compressed," you would:
    a. kardex the order and order the Hemovac
    b. check with the doctor for the amount of pressure
    c. kardex the order only
    d. kardex the order and order a compression machine

18. When ordering "thigh-high Ted hose" for a patient, you must include which of the following?
    a. color of hose
    b. heat setting
    c. size
    d. patient shoe size

19. Sitz bath is the application of warm water to the:
    a. feet
    b. pelvic area
    c. sacral area
    d. whole body

20. A foot cradle is used to:
    a. prevent the top sheet from touching a body part
    b. prevent footdrop
    c. maintain a certain body position
    d. apply heat to a certain body part

21. When transcribing the order "OOB with elastic abd binder," you should include which of the following on the central service department requisition?
    a. waist and hip measurement
    b. chest and hip measurement
    c. no measurement; one size fits all
    d. height and weight

22. In the order "1000 cc 5% D/W KO," KO means:
    a. potassium optional
    b. keep optional
    c. keep open
    d. potassium

23. An infusion pump is used to:
    a. control the amount of IV fluid infused
    b. drain fluid from the surgical site
    c. insert the Foley catheter
    d. suction gastric contents

☑ *ANSWERS AND RATIONALE*

11. **(a)** For the answer, divide 1000 by 125, which tells you each bag will last 8 hours. Three days have a total of 72 hours. Divide 72 by 8, which tells you the total number of bags needed for 3 days. The correct answer is nine 1000-cc bottles. p. 199

12. **(c)** 0.45 normal saline is the solution used most often with the administration of blood. p. 200

13. **(b)** The blood, if not given immediately, must be returned to the blood bank for storage, where safe, even temperature can be maintained. pp. 200, 201

14. **(c)** An LE cell prep is a laboratory test. p. 200

15. **(b)** An intermittent IV line is called a Heplock (heparin lock) pp. 189, 199

16. **(d)** The nasogastric (NG) tube, when used for suctioning purposes, would be connected to wall suction. The tube is inserted through the nose into the stomach. (An NG tube can also be used for tube feeding.) p. 201

17. **(c)** The Hemovac is a disposable wound-suction device usually placed in or near a wound during surgery, so you would kardex the order only. pp. 189, 201

18. **(c)** An order for Ted hose (antiembolism stockings) would require the nurse to measure the patient for proper size. p. 207

19. **(b)** Sitz bath is the application of warm water to the pelvic area. p. 204, 205

20. **(a)** A foot cradle is a metal frame placed on the bed to prevent the top sheet from touching a specified part of the body. p. 206

21. **(a)** Usually the hip and waist measurements are necessary to obtain a correctly fitting binder. p. 207

22. **(c)** KO means "keep open" (or TKO, "to keep open"). When used in IV orders, it is the rate of flow. The usual IV rate is about 50 cc/hr. pp. 190, 199

23. **(a)** An infusion pump is used to control the amount of IV fluid. It is a reusable electric machine obtained from the central service department. pp. 189, 199

NOTES

24. Which of the following orders would require a straight catheter?
    a. intermittent cath irrig 1 hr on, 1 hr clamped
    b. connect cath to continuous Hoffman irrig
    c. cath for residual
    d. irrig cath prn for patency

25. An electrical device used for applying continuous dry heat to the body is called a/an:
    a. Chux pad
    b. K-pad
    c. perineal pad
    d. abdominal pad

26. To void means:
    a. emptying the bladder
    b. leaving a space on the Kardex
    c. omitting a doctor's order
    d. emptying the stomach

27. The order for "TCDB" would be entered in what area on the patient's Kardex form?
    a. vital signs
    b. treatment
    c. respiratory care
    d. activity

28. The term given to blood that is donated for a patient by friends or relatives is:
    a. intraoperative blood cell salvage
    b. autologous blood
    c. donor-specific
    d. occult blood

29. An order reading "Accu-Chek ac and hs" means:
    a. check the glucose level of blood before meals and at bedtime
    b. check acquities before meals and at bedtime
    c. check the glucose level of blood after meals and at bedtime
    d. check acquities after meals and at bedtime

30. An order reading "ORE today" means the patient is to have:
    a. verhead resistive exercises
    b. occupational rehabilitation exercises
    c. outpatient renal endoscopy
    d. oil-retention enema

31. The Jackson-Pratt is a/an:
    a. reusable wound-suction device
    b. electric device used for administering blood
    c. disposable wound-suction device
    d. electric device used for heat application

32. Which of the following doctors' orders would require a consent form?
    a. insertion of a Broviac
    b. Lasix 40 mg IVP stat
    c. convert IV to Heplock with routine saline flushes to keep patent
    d. start IV of D_5LR TKO

33. A Groshong cath is a type of:
    a. straight catheter
    b. indwelling catheter
    c. central venous catheter
    d. intermittent infusion device

34. A doctor's order to use a Port-a-Cath for blood draws would be instructing the nurse to draw blood:
    a. using a special tool called a port-a-cath
    b. from the Heplock
    c. using a portable electronic device called a port-a-cath
    d. from an implanted port

35. If units of blood for two different patients on the unit are ready to be picked up at the same time, the health unit coordinator should:
    a. arrange for two different health care personnel to pick up the units or one to make two trips to pick up each unit separately
    b. ask the lab tech to send the two units of blood by pneumatic tube ASAP
    c. send a health care team member to pick up both units ASAP
    d. leave the desk, go to the blood bank, and pick up both units ASAP

☑ ANSWERS AND RATIONALE

24. **(c)** A straight catheter is used for determining the amount of residual urine in the bladder. It is removed immediately following the procedure. p. 195

25. **(b)** A K-pad is used to apply continuous dry heat to the body. p. 204

26. **(a)** Void means emptying the bladder. p. 189

27. **(b)** Turn, cough, deep breathe (TCDB) is a nursing treatment order and therefore is entered on the treatment area of the Kardex form. pp. 190, 208

28. **(c)** Donor-specific or donor-directed blood is the term used for blood that is donated for a patient by relatives or friends prior to patient need. pp. 189, 200

> Intraoperative blood cell salvage—patient's blood lost during surgery is transfused back into patient
> Autologous blood—the patient's own blood donated previously for transfusion as needed by the patient
> Occult blood—blood that is undetectable to the eye

29. **(a)** Accu-Chek is a type of commercial blood glucose monitor used to check the glucose level of blood; ac means before meals and hs means at bedtime. p. 209

30. **(d)** An oil-retention enema (ORE) is a type of enema. p. 190

31. **(c)** The Jackson-Pratt is a disposable wound-suction device. pp. 201, 203

32. **(a)** The insertion of a Broviac would require a consent form. A Broviac is a type of tunneled catheter, and its insertion is considered a surgical procedure. p. 197

33. **(c)** A Groshong cath is a type of tunneled catheter and is a central venous catheter. p. 197

34. **(d)** Port-a-Cath is a type of port implanted under the skin in the chest wall and may be used by the nurse to draw blood (when ordered by the patient's doctor). pp. 197, 199

35. **(a)** The HUC would arrange for the units to be picked up separately to eliminate the risk of giving the wrong blood to a patient. pp. 200, 201

NOTES

36. Chemotherapy may be administered by means of a:
    a. CBI
    b. CVC
    c. ETS
    d. CMS

37. A chest tube is inserted to:
    a. relieve gas pains
    b. administer medications
    c. reexpand the lungs by removing air or fluid
    d. deliver warm air therapy to lungs

38. Which of the following is used to prevent footdrop of patients who are in bed for long periods?
    a. foot cradle
    b. footboard
    c. air therapy bed
    d. pneumatic hose

39. If a patient's blood specimen were sent to the laboratory for a type and cross-match with a different patient's label affixed to the tube, the specimen would be
    a. processed after the correct identity of the patient was confirmed
    b. discarded and the patient would have to have their blood redrawn
    c. processed after the health unit coordinator went to the laboratory and labeled the tube with the correct patient's label
    d. processed after the RN went to the laboratory and labeled the tube with the correct patient's label

40. For peripheral intravenous therapy, the needle or cannula is inserted:
    a. into a vein in the arm, leg, hand, or foot
    b. through the skin directly into the subclavian or jugular vein
    c. in a vein in the arm and advanced until the tip lies in the superior vena cava
    d. through a small incision made near the subclavian vein

41. A Hickman cath is a type of:
    a. tunneled catheter
    b. percutaneous central venous catheter

c. PICC
d. intermittent infusion device

42. The following doctor's orders require the patient's mental and physical status to be assessed and documented at close and regular intervals.
    a. any type or restraints
    b. pneumatic hose
    c. air therapy bed
    d. Foley catheter

43. The central service department items found on the nursing unit supply closet or C-locker is influenced by:
    a. the popularity of the items (how often doctors ordered them overall)
    b. the amount of the items in stock in the central service department
    c. the specialty of the nursing unit
    d. what the nurses on each nursing unit like to use

44. A penrose drain is used:
    a. when inserting a PICC
    b. during catheterization
    c. when inserting chest tubes
    d. in surgery

45. The abbreviation "ETS" means:
    a. estimated time status
    b. equal to summation
    c. elevated toilet seat
    d. extra time spent

☑ *ANSWERS AND RATIONALE*

36. **(b)** Chemotherapy may be administered by means of a CVC (central venous catheter). p. 199

37. **(c)** A chest tube is inserted to reexpand the lungs by removing air or fluid. p. 204

38. **(b)** A footboard is used to prevent footdrop of patients who are in bed for long periods. pp. 205, 206

39. **(b)** The mislabeled specimen would be discarded and the patient would need to have his or her blood redrawn. Transfusing a patient with an incompatible blood type could be fatal. pp. 200, 201

40. **(a)** Peripheral intravenous therapy would be given by inserting a needle or cannula into a vein in the arm, leg, hand, or foot. Peripheral refers to the blood flow in the extremities of the body. p. 197

41. **(a)** A Hickman cath is a type of tunneled catheter. p. 197

42. **(a)** Use of any type of patient restraint requires a doctor's order and the nurse to assess and document the patient's mental and physical status at close and regular intervals, as prescribed by law and the agency's policies. p. 207

43. **(c)** The type of supplies maintained on the nursing unit supply closet or C-locker would be influenced by the specialty of the unit. For example, an ortho unit would have slings, sand bags, and other items stored in their supply closet or C-locker. p. 191

44. **(d)** A penrose drain is a drain inserted into the patient's surgical wound during surgery. pp. 201, 202

45. **(c)** ETS means extended toilet seat and is used for patients who have difficulty sitting down on a regular toilet seat, such as after total hip replacement surgery. p. 190

TEST-TAKING TIP

Read each stem carefully. Look for key words in the stem such as *first, most important, left or right,* not, except, and so forth.

Dietary Orders

1. A gastrostomy feeding would be administered through which of the following routes?
   a. intravenous
   b. nasal gastric tube
   c. oral
   d. an opening in the abdominal wall

2. Which of the following is a therapeutic diet?
   a. soft
   b. full liquid
   c. low cholesterol
   d. mechanical soft

3. A nurse could choose from which of the following diets when a doctor orders DAT?
   a. clear liquid, full liquid, soft, regular
   b. clear liquid, soft, mechanical soft, 2 g Na
   c. full liquid, soft, pureed, low fat
   d. clear liquid, full liquid, soft, 1200 cal ADA

4. What would a doctor's order for "DAT" require you to do?
   a. send an order to dietary for DAT
   b. check with the patient's nurse
   c. check with the patient
   d. ask the doctor to clarify the order

5. An order for "FF" means that:
   a. all food should be fast fried
   b. extra fluids should be given against patient's will
   c. an IV should be started
   d. extra fluids should be offered to the patient

6. The doctor's order for sips and chips means the patient may have:
   a. sips of water and ice chips
   b. carbonated water and ice chips
   c. Coke and potato chips
   d. tea and ice chips

7. The following is a brand name for a feeding pump:
   a. I-med
   b. Accu-Chek
   c. Kangaroo
   d. Guaiac

8. In the doctor's order "1000-cal ADA diet," ADA means:
   a. adjust diet amount
   b. American Diabetic Association
   c. American Dietetic Association
   d. none of the above

9. In the order "Ensure Plus via bolus feeding 400 cc q 6h," bolus means:
   a. allow the formula to run in by gravity
   b. infuse a small amount of formula over a short time
   c. control the rate of administration
   d. the name of the feeding tube

10. Which of the following is a type of feeding tube?
    a. Osmolite
    b. Jevity
    c. Vivonex-Ten
    d. Dobbhoff

☑ **ANSWERS AND RATIONALE**

1. **(d)** Formula or preparation is fed to the patient through a gastrostomy tube inserted through the abdominal wall into the stomach. pp. 214, 221

2. **(c)** Low cholesterol is a therapeutic diet. Soft, full liquid, and mechanical soft are standard diets with consistency variations. pp. 218, 220

3. **(a)** Clear liquid, full liquid, soft, and regular are choices appropriate for diet as tolerated. pp. 218, 220

4. **(b)** Diet as tolerated (DAT) would require you to check with the patient's nurse to determine the type of diet to order for the patient. pp. 218, 220

5. **(d)** Force fluids (FF) means that extra fluids should be offered to the patient. pp. 215, 222

6. **(a)** Sips and chips means the patient may have sips of water and ice chips. p. 222

7. **(c)** A Kangaroo pump is a brand name for a feeding infusion pump. pp. 214, 221

8. **(b)** ADA stands for the American Diabetic Association. p. 215

9. **(b)** Bolus consists of infusing a small amount of formula over a short time. p. 221

10. **(d)** Dobbhoff is the name of a feeding tube; Osmolite, Jevity, and Vivonex-Ten are types of commercially prepared formulas. p. 221

NOTES

11. What would you order in transcribing the following doctor's order? "Insert Dobbhoff, x-ray for placement. When in proper position, begin via pump, Jevity ½ strength, dilute with H_2O TRA 400 cc/hr for 8 hrs, then 50 cc/hr for 8 hrs, then FS Jevity at 50 cc/hr":
   a. feeding tube, x-ray, Jevity
   b. feeding tube, I-Med, Jevity, x-ray
   c. feeding tube, feeding infusion pump, x-ray, and Jevity
   d. Dobbhoff, Jevity, and x-ray

12. When transcribing a doctor's orders for NPO, sips and chips, allergies, FF, and others, the HUC would:
   a. kardex the information only
   b. send the information to dietary and write the information on the Kardex form
   c. kardex the information and ask the patient's nurse for clarification
   d. call the patient's doctor for clarification of orders

13. Which of the following would cancel out an order for a soft mechanical diet?
   a. limit fluids to 1200 cc/day
   b. 2.5-g Na diet
   c. cl liq diet
   d. NSA

☑ **ANSWERS AND RATIONALE**

11. **(c)** A Dobbhoff (an NG feeding tube), feeding infusion pump, x-ray, and Jevity would be ordered. pp. 221, 222

12. **(b)** Send information to the dietary department and write the information on the Kardex. It is essential that all dietary information be sent to dietary so the necessary adjustments will be made when preparing the patient's trays. p. 217

13. **(c)** An order for a clear liquid diet would change the consistency of the patient's diet and limit fluids to 1200 cc/day; a 2.5-g Na, NSA diet would modify the soft mechanical diet but not cancel it. pp. 218, 220

TEST-TAKING TIP

Read all options carefully before selecting the correct answer. Do not read more into the question.

CHAPTER 13

Medication Orders

1. The process of intravenously infusing carbohydrates, proteins, fats, water, electrolytes, vitamins, and minerals is called:
   a. IVPB
   b. IV push
   c. TPN
   d. PCA

2. A *Broviac* is a type of:
   a. central venous catheter
   b. pacemaker
   c. infusion pump
   d. feeding pump

3. A method by which drugs are administered intravenously in 50 to 100 mL of fluid is called:
   a. intravenous push
   b. intravenous piggyback
   c. intravenous hyperalimentation
   d. parenteral

4. A gelatinous container in which a drug is enclosed is called a/an:
   a. ampoule
   b. tablet
   c. suppository
   d. capsule

5. In which of the following orders is the solution injected under the skin into fat or connective tissue?
   a. Cefadroxil 0.5 g IVPB q 8h
   b. MS 10 mg IM q 4h PRN pain
   c. heparin 10,000 U sub-q stat
   d. Lanoxin 0.5 mg IV push

6. In the order "Timolide ophth 0.25% sol I gtt OS bid," the medication is to be administered in:
   a. the left eye
   b. both eyes
   c. the right eye
   d. the right ear

7. In the order "1000 mL 5% D/W @ KO rate," the mL means:
   a. milliequivalent
   b. milligram
   c. millimeter
   d. milliliter

8. In the order "Maalox 15 cc tid pc," pc means:
   a. before meals
   b. after meals
   c. as needed
   d. with meals

9. A type of medication that relieves pain is called a:
   a. narcotic
   b. tranquilizer
   c. hormone
   d. hypnotic

10. A shortened name given to a drug by a developer is the:
    a. official name
    b. chemical name
    c. generic name
    d. trade name

✔ *ANSWERS AND RATIONALE*

1. **(c)** Total parenteral nutrition (TPN) is the process of intravenously infusing carbohydrates, proteins, fats, water, electrolytes, vitamins, and minerals. p. 228
2. **(a)** A Broviac is a type of long-term central venous catheter. pp. 238–239
3. **(b)** Intravenous piggyback (IVPB) is a method of administering drugs intravenously in 50 to 100 mL of fluid. p. 237
4. **(d)** A capsule is a gelatinous container in which a drug is enclosed. pp. 227 and 236
5. **(c)** Sub-q (also written SQ or SC) is the abbreviation for subcutaneous injection, which is the introduction of a medication under the skin into the fat or connective tissue. pp. 227 and 237
6. **(a)** OS is the abbreviation for left eye. p.228
7. **(d)** mL is the abbreviation for milliliter. p. 227
8. **(b)** pc is the abbreviation for after meals. p. 228
9. **(a)** A narcotic relieves pain and sometimes produces sleep. p. 245
10. **(c)** Generic is the shortened name given to the drug by the developer so that the long chemical name need not be used. p. 234

Generic names of drugs are not capitalized (meperidine). The brand name is always capitalized and may have a trademark symbol (Demerol).

NOTES

11. Which component of a medication order is missing in the doctor's order "Tylenol po q 3h PRN"?
    a. name of drug
    b. dosage of drug
    c. route of administration
    d. frequency of administration

12. In the metric system, the prefix "kilo" is used to:
    a. diminish the basic unit by 100
    b. enlarge the basic unit by 1000
    c. diminish the basic unit by 1000
    d. enlarge the basic unit by 100

13. An order for Vistaril 25 mg IM q 3h for restlessness would be given:
    a. every 3 hours around the clock
    b. every 3 hours until the patient is asleep
    c. only when the patient is restless, every 3 hours
    d. only after verifying with the doctor, in 3-hour intervals when the patient is restless

14. When recopying a patient's MAR, the health unit coordinator notices that a controlled medication with a 3-day stop date has expired. The correct action to take would be to:
    a. discontinue the medication immediately by highlighting it and writing "DC'd" on it
    b. page the patient's doctor or resident to renew the order
    c. stamp the doctor's order sheet with an ink stamp requesting that the order be renewed or discontinued
    d. notify the nurse manager

15. Which of the following is a skin test to diagnose tuberculosis?
    a. TPN
    b. IVPB
    c. IV
    d. PPD

16. Which of the following drugs is a controlled substance?
    a. Synthroid
    b. Dalmane
    c. Ferro-Sequels
    d. Keflex

17. 1000 cc is the same as:
    a. 1000 mg
    b. 1000 mL
    c. 1000 mEq
    d. 1000 L

18. Which of the following is a nonnarcotic analgesic used to lessen pain?
    a. Dilantin
    b. Ibuprofen
    c. Tigan
    d. Maalox

19. Which of the following drugs may be ordered as a treatment for ulcers?
    a. Sonata
    b. Prozac
    c. Librium
    d. Tagamet

20. Which of the following drugs is an antihypertensive drug?
    a. Tagamet
    b. Apresoline
    c. Compazine
    d. Lanoxin

21. Which of the following medications is a diuretic agent that would be given to decrease circulating fluid volume, causing a decrease in pressure demand on the heart?
    a. K-Lor
    b. Lasix
    c. Xanax
    d. digoxin

22. Which of the following is an antiemetic?
    a. Cardizem
    b. Ambien
    c. Cytoxan
    d. Tigan

☑ *ANSWERS AND RATIONALE*

11. **(b)** The dosage of the drug is missing. p. 235
12. **(b)** In the metric system, "kilo" is used to enlarge the basic unit 1000 times. p. 235
13. **(c)** Only when the patient is restless every 3 hours. pp 240–241
14. **(c)** The health unit coordinator should stamp the physician's order sheet with an ink stamp requesting that the order be renewed or discontinued. p. 252
15. **(d)** PPD is a skin test to diagnose tuberculosis. p. 252
16. **(b)** Dalmane is a hypnotic and is a controlled substance. p. 246
17. **(b)** The terms "milliliter" (mL) and "cubic centimeter" (cc) are used interchangeably. p. 227
18. **(b)** Ibuprofen is a nonnarcotic analgesic used to lessen pain. p. 245
19. **(d)** Tagamet (cimetidine) is an antisecretory drug ordered to decrease acid production in the stomach. p. 250
20. **(b)** Apresoline is an antihypertensive that may be ordered to lower blood pressure. p. 249
21. **(b)** Lasix is a diuretic agent that would be given to decrease circulating fluid volume, causing a decrease in pressure demand on the heart. p. 249
22. **(d)** Tigan is an antiemetic. p. 250

NOTES

23. Which of the following drugs is a tranquilizer?
    a. Gantrisin
    b. Xanax
    c. Norflex
    d. Doxidan

24. Which of the following doctor's orders should you question before transcribing?
    a. heparin 5000 U SQ q 8h
    b. Lanoxin 2.5 mg PO qd
    c. Restoril 15 mg PO hs PRN
    d. Keflin 0.5 gm q 6h IV

25. The brand name for digoxin is:
    a. Lovenox
    b. Lasix
    c. Decadron
    d. Lanoxin

26. The generic name for Coumadin is:
    a. Cipro
    b. meperidine
    c. warfarin
    d. diazepam

27. Which of the following groups of drugs has an automatic stop date?
    a. narcotics
    b. antiarthritics
    c. antinauseants
    d. hormones

28. Which of the following is a test for valley fever?
    a. PPD inter today
    b. Cocci 1:100 now
    c. Histoplasmin 0.1 mL today
    d. Give IM placebo now

29. A device used by the patient to control the allowable frequency of his or her pain medication is a/an:
    a. RX
    b. PCN
    c. PCA
    d. CPT

30. An order for Dulcolax is an order for a/an:
    a. narcotic
    b. antianemic
    c. laxative
    d. hormone

31. An order for "Compazine 10 mg IM q 6h N/V" is what kind of an order?
    a. prn
    b. standing
    c. one time
    d. stat

32. An order for "Lomotil tab ī qid for diarrhea" is what kind of an order?
    a. prn
    b. standing
    c. one time
    d. stat

33. An order for "Demerol 50 mg PO now" is what kind of an order?
    a. prn
    b. standing
    c. one time
    d. stat

34. An order for "AquaMephyton 10 mg IM daily × 3 days" is what kind of an order?
    a. prn
    b. standing
    c. one time
    d. short-order series

35. An order for "Lasix 40 mg IM today" would be what kind of an order?
    a. prn
    b. standing
    c. one time
    d. stat

36. The generic name for Lasix is:
    a. Hydrodiuril
    b. furosemide
    c. chlorothiazide
    d. meperidine

37. The generic name for Demerol is:
    a. cimetidine
    b. diazoxide
    c. lidocaine
    d. meperidine

☑ **ANSWERS AND RATIONALE**

23. **(b)** Xanax is a tranquilizer, a drug used to relieve anxiety without causing sleep. p. 246

24. **(b)** The usual adult dose for Lanoxin is 0.125 to 0.25 mg. p. 251

25. **(d)** The brand name for digoxin is Lanoxin. p. 248

26. **(c)** The generic name for Coumadin is warfarin. p. 249

27. **(a)** Narcotics have an automatic stop date. p. 245

28. **(b)** Cocci is a screening test for valley fever. p. 252

29. **(c)** Patient-controlled analgesia (PCA) is a device that allows patients to control the administration of their pain medication. p. 245

30. **(c)** Dulcolax is a laxative. p. 250

31. **(a)** This is a prn (whenever necessary) order. The Compazine would only be given if the patient was nauseated or vomiting (N/V). pp. 245 and 250

32. **(a)** This is a prn order. The qualifying phrase "for diarrhea" indicates that the Lomotil can be given 4 times a day (qid) if the patient has diarrhea. pp. 240 and 250

33. **(d)** Stat means the same as now. p. 242

34. **(d)** This is a short-order series: the AquaMephyton would be given for 3 days as directed and then discontinued. p. 242

35. **(c)** This is a one-time order; the Lasix would be given as directed and then discontinued. pp. 242 and 249

36. **(b)** The generic name for Lasix is furosemide. p. 249

37. **(d)** The generic name for Demerol is meperidine. p. 245

NOTES

38. The generic name for Tylenol is:
    a. furosemide
    b. diazoxide
    c. acetaminophen
    d. desipramine

39. An order for HCTZ is an order for a:
    a. laxative
    b. narcotic
    c. diuretic
    d. antineoplastic

40. An order for "MS" would be given to:
    a. induce urination
    b. relieve pain
    c. reduce cholesterol formation
    d. thin blood

41. To find the usual dosage or the side effects of a medication, you would look in the:
    a. PDR
    b. policy manual
    c. MAR
    d. medical dictionary

42. An order is written on Monday at 0500 for "Lasix 20 mg po q 6h × 5 doses." When would the last dose be given if the first dose is given at 0600?
    a. 6:00 AM on Tuesday
    b. 12:00 midnight on Monday
    c. 12:00 noon on Monday
    d. 12:00 noon on Tuesday

43. An order reads "Donnagel 10 cc PO tid ac." The patient will receive Donnagel:
    a. twice a day before meals
    b. three times a day after meals
    c. twice a day after meals
    d. three times a day before meals

44. A medication to be administered "10 mg IM q 4h" should be given how many times in 24 hours?
    a. three
    b. four
    c. six
    d. eight

45. Lovenox is a medication given to:
    a. relieve severe pain
    b. slow the blood-clotting process
    c. produce or facilitate bowel movements
    d. lower blood pressure

☑ *ANSWERS AND RATIONALE*

RX—treatment, prescription
PCN—penicillin
CPT—chest physical therapy

38. **(c)** The generic name for Tylenol is acetaminophen. p. 245

39. **(c)** Hydrochlorothiazide (HCTZ) is a diuretic. p. 249

40. **(b)** Morphine sulfate (MS) is a narcotic and is given to relieve pain. p. 245

41. **(a)** The *Physician's Desk Reference* (PDR) is where to find usual doses and side effects of medications. pp. 232–233

42. **(a)** The last dose would be given at 6:00 am on Tuesday (q 6h would be 6:00 AM–12:00 noon–6:00 PM–12:00 midnight–6:00 AM for five doses). pp. 240 and 242

43. **(d)** The patient would receive the Donnagel three times a day before meals. p. 240

44. **(c)** The medication would be given six times in 24 hours (24 divided by 4 equals 6). p. 240

45. **(b)** Lovenox is an anticoagulant given to slow the blood-clotting process. p. 249

NOTES

Laboratory Orders and Recording Telephoned Laboratory Results

1. Which of the following specimens is always obtained by the physician?
   a. sputum
   b. pleural fluid
   c. sweat
   d. wound drainage

2. POCT would include which of the following procedures?
   a. Accu-Chek
   b. CMP
   c. T & X-match
   d. CBC

3. An ESR is ordered from which of the following divisions within the laboratory?
   a. hematology
   b. chemistry
   c. microbiology
   d. cytology

4. Which of the following tests is used to determine the oxygen-carrying capacity of the blood and may be used to diagnose anemia?
   a. Hgb
   b. Hct
   c. Diff
   d. Retics

5. Which of the following is used to diagnose lupus erythematosus?
   a. APTT
   b. RBC indices
   c. Retics
   d. LE cell prep

6. Which of the following procedures would be performed to obtain CSF?
   a. biopsy
   b. cervical smear
   c. lumbar puncture
   d. thoracentesis

7. Which of the following assists the physician to determine the dosage of warfarin prescribed in anticoagulant therapy?
   a. PAP
   b. PCV
   c. ESR
   d. PT

8. Which of the following tests usually requires the patient to be fasting?
   a. triglycerides
   b. Lytes
   c. SGOT
   d. LDH

☑ *ANSWERS AND RATIONALE*

1. **(b)** Pleural fluid is obtained by the doctor during a thoracentesis. p. 280
2. **(a)** Accu-Chek is a brand of machine used for blood glucose monitoring and is a point of care testing (done at the bedside). p. 269
3. **(a)** An ESR (erythrocyte sedimentation rate) is a test to determine the rate at which red blood cells settle out of the liquid portion of the blood and is done in the hematology division within the laboratory. p. 271
4. **(a)** Hgb (hemoglobin) is used to determine the oxygen-carrying capacity of the blood. p. 270
5. **(d)** An LE cell prep is used to diagnose lupus erythematosus. p. 271
6. **(c)** A lumbar puncture would be performed to obtain CSF (cerebral spinal fluid). p. 281
7. **(d)** A PT (prothrombin time) measures the clotting ability of the blood and is used to monitor the dosages of warfarin. p. 269
8. **(a)** An order for triglycerides requires the patient to be fasting. p. 274, Table 14–1

NOTES

9. You are transcribing a doctor's order for electrolytes, which would include which of the following?
   a. Na, K, Cl, CO_2
   b. Na, CK, K, CO_2
   c. Na, K, Cl, Ca
   d. K, Cl, CO_2, LDH

10. Which of the following tests may be used to diagnose and/or monitor diabetes?
    a. BUN
    b. AST
    c. CPK
    d. FBS

11. The health unit coordinator would be required to consult the patient's nurse to coordinate which of the following physicians' orders?
    a. CBC and CMP—call if K is below 3.5
    b. T & C 2 units packed cells for transfusion today
    c. theophylline peak and trough around third dose
    d. clean-catch urine for C & S

12. Which of the following are cardiac enzymes and may be ordered when a myocardial infarction is suspected?
    a. AST, CPK, LDH
    b. ALT, CPK, LDH
    c. GTT, CPK, AST
    d. AST, CPK, ALT

13. Which of the following tests is useful in diagnosing diseases that affect kidney function?
    a. Bili
    b. BUN
    c. TIBC
    d. LDH

14. You have just received the following laboratory test values by telephone. Which is a critical value and should be brought to the nurse's attention immediately?
    a. WBC is 8500
    b. K is 4.8
    c. FBS is 575
    d. PT is 14 seconds

15. For the doctor's order "2-hr PPBS," it is your responsibility to:
    a. notify the lab of the time the patient last voided
    b. notify the lab when the patient has finished eating
    c. notify the lab when the patient received his or her food tray
    d. notify the lab when the patient requests to have the test done

16. You would order a serum creatinine test from which of the following laboratory divisions?
    a. serology
    b. urinalysis
    c. hematology
    d. chemistry

17. Which of the following laboratory tests is used to guide antibiotic treatment?
    a. Gram stain
    b. mycology studies
    c. AFB culture
    d. culture and sensitivity

18. You would order an "RA factor" from which of the following laboratory divisions?
    a. serology
    b. bacteriology
    c. hematology
    d. chemistry

19. The order "cryoprecipitate 1 unit" would be ordered from which of the following laboratory divisions?
    a. hematology
    b. chemistry
    c. bacteriology
    d. blood bank

20. Which of the following is a blood bank order?
    a. Coombs' test
    b. AST
    c. ASO titer
    d. BNP

21. Which of the following tests would be performed with an order for a unit of PC?
    a. PCV
    b. Coombs test
    c. PTT
    d. T & X-match

☑ **ANSWERS AND RATIONALE**

9. **(a)** Sodium (Na), potassium (K), chloride (Cl), and carbon dioxide (CO_2) make up electrolytes. p. 273

10. **(d)** FBS (fasting blood sugar) determines the amount of sugar in the bloodstream after the patient has not eaten for 8 to 10 hours and is used to diagnose and/or monitor diabetes. p. 273

11. **(c)** The patient's nurse would need to be consulted to determine when the third dose of theophylline will be given. The test will be ordered a half-hour before and an hour after the patient receives the medication (times may vary among hospitals). p. 274

12. **(a)** AST, CPK, and LDH are the cardiac enzymes. p. 272

13. **(b)** BUN (blood urea nitrogen) is used to diagnose diseases affecting the kidney. p. 273

14. **(c)** The normal FBS value is 70 to 120; a fasting blood sugar of 575 should be brought to the nurse's attention immediately. p. 273

15. **(b)** The laboratory must be notified when the patient has finished eating so the blood can be drawn 2 hours after the patient has finished eating. p. 274

A 2-hour postprandial blood sugar is a test performed to determine the patient's response to carbohydrate intake. The blood specimen must be drawn 2 hours after the patient has finished eating. Nursing personnel may be responsible for drawing the patient's blood in many hospitals.

16. **(d)** A serum creatinine test is ordered from the chemistry division of the laboratory. p. 273

17. **(d)** A culture and sensitivity is used to guide antibiotic treatment. p. 276

18. **(a)** An RA factor, a test for rheumatoid arthritis, is ordered from the serology division of the laboratory. p. 278

19. **(d)** A unit of cryoprecipitate is ordered from the blood bank within the laboratory. p. 279

20. **(a)** A Coombs' test also called the direct antiglobulin test. DAT is a blood bank order. p. 279

A positive Coombs' test is found in hemolytic disease of the newborn, hemolytic transfusion reactions, and acquired hemolytic anemia. The indirect Coombs' test detects the presence of antibodies to red blood cell antigens. This test is valuable in detecting the presence of anti-Rh antibodies in the serum of a pregnant woman before delivery.

21. **(d)** A T & C (type and crossmatch) must be done to obtain a unit of packed cells (PC). p. 278

NOTES

22. Which of the following studies is used by a physician to aid in the diagnosis of diabetes?
    a. 6-hour GTT
    b. AST
    c. TIBC
    d. creatinine clearance

23. The symbol representing iron is:
    a. Ir
    b. Fi
    c. Fe
    d. In

24. Which of the following is a chemistry panel consisting of fourteen chemistry tests?
    a. BMP
    b. CMP
    c. BNP
    d. CPK

25. Which of the following tests would be performed in toxicology?
    a. serum osmolality
    b. digoxin level
    c. troponin
    d. TSH

26. Which of the following diet orders would be appropriate for a patient who is to be "fasting"?
    a. DAT
    b. full liq
    c. water only
    d. NPO

27. Which of the following tests is a count of immature red blood cells?
    a. Diff
    b. Hgb
    c. Retics
    d. platelets

28. Which of the following tests is used for the diagnosis of infection?
    a. WBC
    b. RBC
    c. Hgb
    d. Plts

29. Which of the following tests would be done to diagnose a thyroid problem?
    a. TIBC
    b. triglycerides
    c. uric acid
    d. TSH

30. Which of the following lab tests would require the patient to sign a consent form prior to it being ordered?
    a. anti-OKT$_3$ antibody level
    b. CEA
    c. HIVB$_{24}$Ag
    d. FTA

31. What procedure would be done to obtain a bone marrow specimen?
    a. amniocentesis
    b. sternal puncture
    c. lumbar puncture
    d. biopsy

32. Which of the following lab tests would require the health unit coordinator to send an NPO order to the dietary department?
    a. FBS
    b. 6-hour GTT
    c. cholesterol
    d. triglycerides

33. A PSA is a laboratory test to assist in the diagnosis of:
    a. kidney disease
    b. prostate cancer
    c. breast cancer
    d. pancreatic cancer

34. An "RPR" is a test performed to diagnose:
    a. gout
    b. syphilis
    c. anemia
    d. diabetes

35. A test performed to diagnose acute myocardial infarction from a few hours' onset to as long as 120 hours is a/an:
    a. ANA
    b. CEA
    c. troponin
    d. RDW

36. A test performed to assess treatment of liver, colon, or pancreatic cancer is a/an:
    a. CEA
    b. ANA
    c. FTA
    d. complement fixation titer

☑ **ANSWERS AND RATIONALE**

22. **(a)** A 6-hour GTT (glucose tolerance test) is performed to determine abnormalities in glucose metabolism and is used to aid in the diagnosis of diabetes. p. 273

> For a 6-hour glucose tolerance test, the patient is in a fasting state. The test is performed over 6 hours. The patient has an FBS (fasting blood sugar) drawn to establish baseline data and then is given a large amount of glucose solution to drink. Timed blood and urine specimens are taken. At the completion of the test, all urine is sent to the laboratory.

23. **(c)** Fe is the symbol for iron. p. 261
24. **(b)** A CMP comprehensive metabolic chemistry panel consists of 14 chemistry tests. p. 273
25. **(b)** A digoxin level is done in toxicology. p. 274
26. **(c)** Fasting means the patient may have water; NPO means nothing by mouth. p. 271
27. **(c)** Reticulocytes (Retics) are the count of immature red blood cells, which determines bone marrow activity. This test is often used in the diagnosis of anemia. p. 271
28. **(a)** White blood cells (WBCs; leukocytes) fight disease-causing organisms. p. 271
29. **(d)** The thyroid-stimulating hormone (TSH) test would be done to diagnose a thyroid problem. p. 274
30. **(c)** Human immunodeficiency virus (HIV) is the virus that causes AIDS (acquired immunodeficiency syndrome) and the test to detect the virus, $HIVB_{24}Ag$, would require the patient to sign a consent prior to it being performed. p. 278
31. **(b)** A sternal puncture would be done to obtain bone marrow. p. 267
32. **(b)** A 6-hour GTT (glucose tolerance test) requires that the dietary department be notified so a food tray would not be delivered to the patient. The other tests would be completed prior to breakfast time. p. 273
33. **(b)** A prostatic specific antigen (PSA) is a laboratory test to assist in the diagnosis of prostate cancer. p. 273
34. **(b)** Syphilis may be diagnosed by performing a rapid plasma reagin (RPR). This test is also called a VDRL (Venereal Disease Research Laboratory). p. 278
35. **(c)** Troponin is a test performed to diagnose acute myocardial infarction. p. 274
36. **(a)** An elevated level of CEA (carcinoembryonic antigen) may indicate liver, colon, or pancreatic cancer. The CEA level is also used to assess the treatment of these conditions. p. 278

NOTES

37. When an order for "guaiac all stools" is written, the purpose is to detect:
    a. sodium
    b. fat
    c. occult blood
    d. sugar

38. Which of the following procedures requires the patient to sign a consent form?
    a. 1 unit cryoprecipitate
    b. EBV panel
    c. CMV culture
    d. PAP smear

39. A CBC would include which of the following tests?
    a. WBC/Diff, RBC, PT, ESR
    b. WBC/Diff, RBC, Hgb, Hct
    c. WBC/Diff, PCV, ESR, APIT
    d. WBC/Diff, RBC, Na, K

40. An order for a 24-hour urine specimen would require you to order a:
    a. catheter tray from SPD
    b. container from the lab
    c. nonretention catheter from SPD
    d. container from SPD

41. An order for a sterile urine specimen would be obtained by which of the following methods?
    a. clean catch
    b. midstream
    c. catheterization
    d. voided

42. Which of the following specimens should be hand carried and never sent to the laboratory via tube system?
    a. CSF
    b. blood
    c. stool
    d. sputum

43. An order written by a doctor for "creatinine" may be interpreted by the health unit coordinator as an order for a serum creatinine because:
    a. the doctor did not specify any other specimen
    b. creatinine is not a test performed on any other specimen
    c. all tests are performed on serum
    d. the doctor would need to be called to verify the order

44. The division of the laboratory that studies immunologic substances is:
    a. chemistry
    b. serology
    c. hematology
    d. microbiology

45. Which of the following items are required to be handwritten on a patient ID label affixed to a laboratory specimen?
    a. date, time, and the initials of the person who collected the specimen
    b. the test to be performed on the specimen
    c. the name of the doctor who ordered the test
    d. date, time, and the initials of the person completing the requisition

46. Uric acid levels are used principally to diagnose:
    a. diabetes
    b. gout
    c. pancreatic cancer
    d. rheumatoid arthritis

47. The health unit coordinator can avoid errors when receiving telephoned laboratory results by:
    a. writing them first in pencil
    b. reading the values back to the person reporting them
    c. carefully checking them before reporting them to the nurse
    d. asking someone to listen on another phone

☑ ANSWERS AND RATIONALE

37. **(c)** The purpose of an order for "guaiac all stools" is to detect occult (hidden) blood. pp. 260, 269

38. **(a)** Cryoprecipitate is a blood product for transfusion and would need a signed consent by the patient. p. 279

39. **(b)** A WBC/Diff (white blood cell count with differential), RBC (red blood cell count), Hgb (hemoglobin), and Hct (hematocrit) are included in a CBC. p. 270

40. **(b)** An order for a 24-hour urine specimen would require you to order a container from the lab. Some specimens, such as a 24-hour urine specimen, are kept for a period of time; therefore, a preservative may be added to the collection bottle before it is sent to the unit. p. 271

41. **(c)** Catheterization is required to obtain a sterile urine sample. p. 280

42. **(a)** CSF (cerebrospinal fluid) is obtained by an invasive procedure (lumbar puncture), and therefore must be hand carried to the laboratory. p. 281

43. **(a)** The doctor did not specify any other specimen (i.e., urine creatinine). Most lab tests that do not specify another specimen are performed on serum. Often the doctor will write *serum creatinine.* pp. 266, 267

44. **(b)** Serology performs tests that study diseases of the immune system. pp. 276, 277

45. **(a)** The date, time, and the initials of the person who collected the specimen are required to be handwritten on the patient ID label affixed to the specimen. p. 267

46. **(b)** Uric acid levels are used principally to diagnose gout. p. 274

47. **(b)** Reading values back to the person reporting them will reduce risk of errors in receiving telephoned laboratory results. p. 281

NOTES

Diagnostic Imaging Orders

1. Contrast media are used in diagnostic imaging procedures to:
   a. differentiate between bone structures
   b. clear the patient's intestinal tract
   c. increase the contrast in different body tissue densities
   d. ensure that the patient does not feel any discomfort

2. The doctor has ordered a "BE, UGI, and US of ABD." Which one should be scheduled first?
   a. UGI
   b. US of ABD
   c. BE
   d. it doesn't matter

3. A study that uses a device to record views of selected levels of the body by means of a computer and may be done with or without a contrast medium is a:
   a. fluoroscopy
   b. CT scan
   c. lymphangiogram
   d. MUGA scan

4. A BE is a procedure performed to visualize the:
   a. renal pelvis
   b. small intestine
   c. upper gastrointestinal area
   d. large intestine

5. "On call" medication may be defined as medication that:
   a. is given when the patient requests it
   b. requires that the doctor be called before giving it
   c. requires the nurse to call the department performing the procedure on the patient for a medication order
   d. requires the nurse to give a previously ordered medication when the department performing a procedure calls the nursing station with instructions to do so

6. The doctor's orders include BE, UGI, and a total bone scan. Which procedure would you schedule to be done first?
   a. total bone scan
   b. BE
   c. it doesn't matter
   d. UGI

7. The procedure used to outline the kidney, renal pelvis, ureters, and urinary bladder is called a/an:
   a. IVU
   b. BE
   c. MUGA scan
   d. UGI

8. A procedure that requires the nursing staff to prepare the patient before the procedure is a/an:
   a. KUB
   b. IVU
   c. chest x-ray
   d. angiogram

☑ *ANSWERS AND RATIONALE*

1. **(c)** Because there is little difference in density between certain organs and blood vessels, contrast media are used to increase the contrast. pp. 289, 295

2. **(b)** Abdominal studies using ultrasound (US) should precede studies using barium, because barium in specific parts of the body may obscure the portion of the body being studied by US. p. 295

3. **(c)** Computerized tomography (CT) records and displays selected cross-sectional images of any body part and may be ordered with or without contrast media. p. 301

4. **(d)** A BE (barium enema) is a procedure used to visualize the large intestine. p. 298

5. **(d)** "On call" medications are prescribed by the doctor to be given on call prior to the procedure. pp. 289, 299

6. **(a)** The total bone scan should be done first because the barium used to perform a BE and a UGI would obscure the bone scan. p. 295

7. **(a)** An IVU (intravenous urogram; may also be called an IVP, or intravenous pyelogram) outlines the kidneys, renal pelvis, ureters, and urinary bladder. p. 296

8. **(b)** Preparation of the patient is necessary for an intravenous urogram (UGI). p. 296

NOTES

9. Which of the following schedules of diagnostic studies is incorrect?
   a. (1) US of pelvis; (2) BE; (3)UGI
   b. (1) IVP; (2) GB; (3) BE; (4) UGI
   c. (1) BE; (2) UGI; (3) liver and spleen scan
   d. (1) Total bone scan; (2) IVP; (3) BE

10. The abbreviation "PA" used with an x-ray order requires the radiographer to position the patient:
    a. either standing or lying on his or her back (supine) with the x-ray machine placed in front of the patient
    b. on his or her side
    c. lying halfway on his or her side
    d. either standing or lying on his or her stomach (prone) with the x-ray machine aimed at the back of the patient

11. An order for an L-S spine x-ray is an order for the:
    a. low sacral area
    b. lumbosacral area
    c. lateral-sacral area
    d. left sacral area

12. An order written for a KUB is a request for an x-ray of the:
    a. kidneys, ureters, and bladder
    b. kidneys, urethra, and bladder
    c. kidneys, ureter, and bile duct
    d. kidneys, uterus, and bladder

13. Fluoroscopy is:
    a. the observation of deep body structures made visible by use of a TV screen
    b. a technique that uses high-frequency sound waves to create an image of body organs
    c. the image produced when the concentration of radionuclide in an organ is photographed
    d. a measurement and record of heat energy emanating from the body surface

14. Which of the following procedures requires the patient to drink sufficient water to fill the bladder before being sent to the diagnostic imaging department?
    a. cholecystogram
    b. retrograde pyelogram
    c. renal ultrasound
    d. intravenous urogram

15. A procedure using a powerful magnetic field and in which bones do not obscure the images as they do in x-rays is a/an:
    a. MRI
    b. nuclear medicine
    c. CT scan
    d. fluoroscopy

16. Which of the following procedures requires contrast medium?
    a. arteriogram
    b. mammogram
    c. KUB
    d. skull series

17. An order for a CT scan of the L-S spine is performed in which of the following divisions of medical imaging?
    a. nuclear medicine
    b. computerized tomography
    c. endoscopy
    d. special x-ray procedures

18. A scan of the biliary tract (gallbladder) is called a:
    a. gallium scan
    b. thallium scan
    c. cholangiogram
    d. DISIDA scan

19. Which of the following divisions of radiology would use radiopharmaceuticals (isotopes) to determine the functioning capacity of organs?
    a. magnetic resonance imaging
    b. nuclear medicine
    c. computerized tomography
    d. ultrasound

20. A lung perfusion-ventilation study is done in which of the following areas?
    a. cardiology
    b. pulmonary function
    c. nuclear medicine
    d. computerized tomography

21. Which of the following procedures requires a signed consent form by the patient?
    a. mammogram
    b. arthrogram
    c. US of the GB
    d. tomogram of the lung

☑ *ANSWERS AND RATIONALE*

9. **(c)** The presence of barium would obscure visualization of the liver and spleen. Nuclear medicine studies should be done prior to barium studies for this reason. p. 295

10. **(d)** PA (posterior-anterior) requires the radiographer to have the patient standing or lying on his or her stomach (prone) with the x-ray machine aimed at the back of the patient. p. 292

11. **(b)** L-S stands for lumbosacral. p. 290

12. **(a)** KUB stands for kidneys, ureters, and bladder. p. 290

13. **(a)** Fluoroscopy is the observation of deep body structures made visible by use of a TV screen. p. 289

14. **(c)** The patient will be given a certain amount of water to drink and will be instructed not to void before a renal ultrasound. p. 303

15. **(a)** MRI (magnetic resonance imaging) studies are done on selected areas of the body. A computer records cross-sectional images of the part being studied. p. 303

16. **(a)** An arteriogram requires an injection of contrast medium. p. 299

17. **(b)** A CT scan is performed in the computerized tomography division of medical imaging. p. 301

18. **(d)** A DISIDA scan, a nuclear medicine procedure, is a scan of the biliary tract. p. 306

19. **(b)** The nuclear medicine division would use radiopharmaceuticals (isotopes). p. 305

20. **(c)** Lung perfusion-ventilation is a nuclear medicine study done to diagnose embolisms. p. 306

21. **(b)** An arthrogram is an invasive procedure and requires a signed patient consent form. p. 299

NOTES

22. An x-ray of the cerebral vascular structures is called a cerebral:
    a. myelogram
    b. PET scan
    c. angiogram
    d. venogram

23. A hysterosalpingogram is an x-ray of which of the following organs?
    a. body tissues and salivary ducts
    b. uterus and ovaries
    c. ovaries and surrounding tissues
    d. uterus and fallopian tubes

24. The abbreviation "LLQ" means:
    a. low-level quota
    b. left lobe quadrant
    c. left lower quadrant
    d. left lumbar quadrant

25. A "routine preparation" is one that:
    a. the patient routinely takes at home on a daily basis
    b. is given for all x-ray procedures
    c. is suggested by the radiologist to prepare the patient for a diagnostic imaging study
    d. is a preparation routinely given on a particular nursing unit

26. An order for "SBFT" is:
    a. special bowel follow-through
    b. special bladder fluoroscopy therapy
    c. small bowel follow-through
    d. small bowel fluoroscopy transfer

27. An order for a MUGA scan would require you to send a requisition to:
    a. CT scanning
    b. nuclear medicine
    c. MRI
    d. special procedures

28. Which of the following items would need to be noted on a diagnostic imaging requisition?
    a. time procedure is to be done
    b. dates of patient's previous admissions
    c. reason for the procedure
    d. patient's nationality

29. Which of the following would be important to note on a requisition when ordering an x-ray procedure: The patient is:
    a. Catholic
    b. HIV positive
    c. a VIP
    d. hearing impaired

30. Which of the following facts about the patient would need to be noted on a diagnostic imaging requisition:
    a. patient may be subject to seizures
    b. patient is taking antibiotics
    c. patient is HIV positive
    d. patient is Asian

31. A patient who has a pacemaker should not be scheduled for which of the following procedures?
    a. bone scan
    b. MRI of left humerus
    c. CT of the chest
    d. myelography

32. An order is written for an "x-ray of rt femur" on a patient admitted with a diagnosis of cholelithiasis. There is no clinical indication given for the x-ray. The health unit coordinator would:
    a. order the x-ray and note that there was no reason given
    b. fill in the admitting diagnosis for the reason for the x-ray
    c. leave the reason for the x-ray blank
    d. call the doctor who wrote the order and ask the reason for the x-ray

33. Which of the following procedures would require the health unit coordinator to obtain a form for the patient's nurse to complete ensuring that the patient does not have a pacemaker, cerebral aneurysm clips, or any electrically, magnetically, or mechanically activated implants?
    a. CT of the brain
    b. tomogram of rt lung
    c. renal US
    d. MRI rt knee

☑ *ANSWERS AND RATIONALE*

22. **(c)** A cerebral angiogram is an x-ray of the cerebral vascular structures. p. 299

23. **(d)** A hysterosalpingogram is an x-ray of the uterus and fallopian tubes. p. 300

24. **(c)** LLQ means left lower quadrant. p. 290

25. **(c)** A "routine preparation" is one suggested by the radiologist. pp. 290, 295

26. **(c)** "SBFT" means small bowel follow-through. pp. 290, 298

27. **(b)** The requisition would be sent to nuclear medicine; a MUGA scan is a multigated angiogram, a type of cardiac scan. p. 306

28. **(c)** The reason for the procedure (clinical indication) must be noted on the diagnostic imaging requisition. p. 291

29. **(d)** It would be important to note that the patient is hearing impaired. p. 291

30. **(a)** It is important to note that the patient is subject to seizures on the diagnostic imaging requisition. p. 291

31. **(b)** Due to the strength of the magnet and the radiofrequency waves, MRI contraindications exist for patients with pacemakers, cerebral aneurysm clips, or any electrically, magnetically, or mechanically activated implants. p. 303

32. **(d)** Call the doctor who wrote the order and ask the reason for the x-ray. It is essential for the diagnostic imaging department to know the reason for the procedure. (Other options include checking the doctor's progress notes or asking the patient's nurse.) pp. 291, 292

33. **(d)** An "MRI rt knee" order would require the patient's nurse to complete a form ensuring that the patient does not have a pacemaker, cerebral aneurysm clips, or any electrically, magnetically, or mechanically activated implants due to the powerful magnet and the radiofrequency waves used during the procedure. p. 303

NOTES

34. A procedure performed by nuclear medicine to obtain information about blood flow to the myocardium is a:
   a. lung perfusion-ventilation study
   b. PET scan
   c. thallium stress scan
   d. DISIDA scan

35. A procedure performed to locate the primary site of cancer, as well as to detect an abscess, is a:
   a. MUGA scan
   b. thallium stress test
   c. gallium scan
   d. PET

☑ **ANSWERS AND RATIONALE**

34. **(b)** A PET (positron emission tomography) scan is used to obtain information about blood flow in the myocardium. p. 306

35. **(c)** A gallium scan is performed to locate the primary site of cancer, as well as to detect an abscess. p. 306

NOTES

Pg 151 ___ Chapt 12

Advance diet

Amb c̄ Asst.

Heart MEDS
Isoenzymz
TROPRO
LDL
CPK

Amb-TB test.
Icelation

PCA

Other Diagnostic Studies

1. In the order "ABG on RA" RA stands for:
   a. right arm
   b. rotating air
   c. room air
   d. right atrium

2. A transesophageal electrocardiogram is ordered from which of the following hospital departments?
   a. diagnostic imaging
   b. cardiovascular diagnostics
   c. neurodiagnostics
   d. respiratory

3. An order for a CBG is a request for a:
   a. capillary blood gas
   b. complete blood gas
   c. cell blood gas
   d. complete blood gestation

4. Which of the following medications is to be noted when ordering an ABG?
   a. Lasix
   b. Lipitor
   c. Heparin
   d. Motrin

5. You would order a 2D M-mode echo from which of the following hospital departments?
   a. neurodiagnostics
   b. diagnostic imaging
   c. respiratory care
   d. cardiovascular diagnostics

6. A doctor's order for IPG–rt leg would require the health unit coordinator to send a requisition to which of the following departments?
   a. diagnostic imaging
   b. endoscopy
   c. neurodiagnostics
   d. cardiovascular diagnostics

7. The doctor's order for a stress test refers to a:
   a. psychological test
   b. treadmill test
   c. physical therapy exercise
   d. gastroenterology test

8. Which of the following medications is noted when ordering an EKG?
   a. Lanoxin
   b. Phenergan
   c. Benadryl
   d. Synthroid

9. A balloon-tipped catheter inserted through the subclavian vein into the right side of the heart through the right ventricle and into a branch of the pulmonary artery is called a:
   a. pacemaker
   b. Swan-Ganz catheter
   c. flexible radiopaque catheter
   d. Foley catheter

☑ *ANSWERS AND RATIONALE*

1. **(c)** RA stands for room air, and in the order ABG (arterial blood gases) on RA, the patient must not be on oxygen therapy. pp. 313, 324

2. **(b)** A transesophageal electrocardiogram examines cardiac function and structure with an ultrasound transducer placed in the esophagus. It is a cardiovascular study. p. 317

3. **(a)** CBG is the abbreviation for capillary blood gas. p. 324

4. **(c)** Heparin, an anticoagulant, is noted when ordering an ABG to indicate the possibility of excessive bleeding during the puncturing of the artery to obtain the specimen. p. 324

5. **(d)** A 2D M-mode echo is a cardiovascular study. p. 317

6. **(d)** An IPG (impedance plethysmography) shows changes in the blood volume and would require the health unit coordinator to send a requisition to cardiovascular diagnostics. p. 317

7. **(b)** A stress test refers to a treadmill procedure. p. 317

8. **(a)** Lanoxin, a cardiac medication, is noted when ordering an EKG (electrocardiogram). p. 315

9. **(b)** A Swan-Ganz catheter is a balloon-tipped catheter usually inserted by a doctor in the intensive care unit. p. 318

NOTES

10. An order for an ambulatory ECG, which requires the patient to keep a 24-hour diary of activities performed while wearing an ECG tape recorder, would be ordered from which of the following hospital departments?
    a. cardiovascular diagnostics
    b. neurodiagnostics
    c. central service
    d. respiratory

11. Which of the following is an invasive procedure and therefore requires you to prepare a consent form?
    a. cardiac catheterization
    b. EMG
    c. treadmill stress test
    d. 2D M-mode echo

12. Doppler flow studies are ordered by the doctor to determine:
    a. air flow through the lungs
    b. gastric acidity
    c. blood flow within blood vessels
    d. malabsorption of fat

13. Endoscopy is a generic term used to indicate:
    a. an artificial opening into an organ
    b. visual examination of a body cavity
    c. removal of an organ
    d. visual examination of an eye

14. Which of the following procedures would have to be scheduled *after* a sigmoidoscopy?
    a. EEG
    b. BE
    c. VCG
    d. SVN

15. A gastroscopy is a procedure used to:
    a. visualize the interior of the stomach
    b. measure gastric acidity
    c. create an artificial opening into the stomach
    d. visualize the intestines

16. OSA is an abbreviation meaning:
    a. occupational safety assessment
    b. ocular saturation assessment
    c. orthopedic skeletal alignment
    d. obstructive sleep apnea

17. A procedure performed to measure a patient's lung capacity for air is called a/an:
    a. incentive spirometry
    b. ABG on RA
    c. spirometry
    d. CBG

18. A BAER is a procedure used to record:
    a. breathing capabilities
    b. response to stimulation of a peripheral nerve
    c. hearing response
    d. involuntary eye movements

19. A SEP is a procedure used to record:
    a. breathing capabilities
    b. response to stimulation of a peripheral nerve
    c. hearing response
    d. involuntary eye movements

20. An ENG would be ordered from which of the following hospital departments?
    a. endoscopy
    b. neurodiagnostics
    c. respiratory
    d. cardiovascular diagnostics

21. The following diagnostic procedure would be coordinated with the neurodiagnostic department and the cardiovascular department:
    a. impedance plethysmography study
    b. carotid phonoangiography
    c. electrophysiological study
    d. Persantine stress test

22. A procedure done to inspect the common bile duct, biliary tract, and pancreatic duct by inserting a catheter through an endoscope is called a/an:
    a. EGD
    b. ERCP
    c. PTHC
    d. EEG

23. Which of the following procedures would require a consent form?
    a. cardiac monitor
    b. Doppler flow studies
    c. sigmoidoscopy
    d. evoked potentials

☑ *ANSWERS AND RATIONALE*

10. **(a)** Cardiovascular diagnostics would place a Holter monitor, which produces an ambulatory electrocardiogram. p. 317

11. **(a)** A cardiac catheterization requires entry into the body by placing a catheter into a blood vessel and the heart, and therefore is an invasive procedure. p. 318

12. **(c)** Doppler flow studies show flow changes caused by changes within the blood vessels. p. 317

13. **(b)** Endoscopy indicates the visual examination of a body cavity or hollow organ. p. 320

14. **(b)** A BE (barium enema) involves the filling of the colon with barium, making it impossible to visualize the interior of the sigmoid colon. p. 321

15. **(a)** Gastroscopy is the visual examination of the interior of the stomach by means of a gastroscope. p. 321

16. **(d)** OSA is an abbreviation for obstructive sleep apnea. pp. 313, 325

17. **(c)** Spirometry is a procedure performed to measure a patient's lung capacity for air. pp. 324, 325

18. **(c)** A BAER (brain stem auditory evoked response), also called AER, is used to record hearing response. pp. 313, 320

19. **(b)** A SEP (somatosensory evoked potentials) is performed by neurodiagnostics to monitor neurologic function. pp. 313, 320

20. **(b)** An ENG (electronystagmography) is done by placing electrodes near the patient's eyes to record involuntary eye movements. pp. 313, 320

21. **(d)** A Persantine stress test is a two-step process involving the neurodiagnostics department and the cardiovascular department. p. 318

22. **(b)** This procedure is called an ERCP (endoscopic retrograde cholangiopancreatography). pp. 313, 321

23. **(c)** A sigmoidoscopy is a visual examination of the sigmoid colon and would require a consent form. p. 321

NOTES

24. Which of the following procedures would
    be performed in the endoscopy
    department?
    a. EGD
    b. AER
    c. IPG
    d. VEP

ANSWERS AND RATIONALE

24. **(a)** An EGD (esophagogastroduodenoscopy) is the visual examination of the upper gastrointestinal tract and would be performed in the endoscopy department. p. 321

NOTES

Treatment Orders

1. Buck's traction is used to treat fractures of the:
   a. humerus
   b. pelvic bone
   c. cervical vertebra
   d. hip or knee

2. Two main types of traction used in hospitals include:
   a. swinging and pull
   b. skeletal and skin
   c. splint and implanted
   d. straight and elevated

3. An order for an induced sputum specimen would require the health unit coordinator to:
   a. inform the patient's resident
   b. send the request to the laboratory
   c. inform the patient's nurse to take a sputum cup in to the patient
   d. send the request to the respiratory care department

4. An incentive spirometry is a:
   a. technique used postoperatively to encourage patients to breathe deeply
   b. measurement of a patient's lung capacity for air
   c. procedure done to push air into the lungs during inspiration
   d. heated mist for the patient to breathe in

5. You would order ADL from which of the following departments?
   a. dietary
   b. physical therapy
   c. occupational therapy
   d. respiratory care

6. You would order TENS from which of the following hospital departments?
   a. occupational therapy
   b. physical therapy
   c. central service
   d. cardiovascular studies

7. The meaning of the abbreviation CPM is:
   a. complete patient message
   b. central pleural myogram
   c. complete posture mechanics
   d. continuous passive motion

8. Which of the following is used for hydrotherapy?
   a. diathermy
   b. range of motion
   c. aerosol
   d. whirlpool

9. You would order "ultrasound and massage to lower back" from which of the following departments?
   a. ultrasound
   b. physical therapy
   c. radiology
   d. respiratory care

10. A doctor's order for an "ABG 1 hour $\bar{p}$ increasing O_2 to 4 L/m" would require the health unit coordinator to:
    a. order an oxygen setup from respiratory
    b. order an ABG only
    c. go to the patient's room to adjust the O_2 flow rate
    d. notify the patient's nurse and order the ABG with the specific directions

✔ *ANSWERS AND RATIONALE*

1. **(d)** Buck's traction is used to treat hip or knee fractures/disorders p. 337
2. **(d)** Skeletal traction and skin traction are two main types of traction used in hospitals. p. 336
3. **(d)** An induced-sputum specimen is collected by the respiratory department. p. 340
4. **(a)** Incentive spirometry is a technique used postoperatively to encourage the patient to deep breathe. The order would be sent to the respiratory department. p. 341
5. **(c)** ADL (activities of daily living) is ordered from the occupational therapy department. pp. 331, 346
6. **(b)** TENS (transcutaneous electrical nerve stimulation) is used to control pain and is carried out by the physical therapy department. pp. 331, 345
7. **(d)** CPM is the abbreviation for continuous passive motion and is a type of physical therapy done on a machine after joint replacement surgery. pp. 331, 344
8. **(d)** A whirlpool is used by the physical therapy department for hydrotherapy. pp. 343, 344
9. **(b)** "Ultrasound and massage" is a heat treatment administered by the physical therapy department. p. 345
10. **(d)** "ABG 1 hour $\bar{c}$ increasing O_2 to 4 L/m" is not a new oxygen order. The order indicates that the ABG is to be done 1 hour after the oxygen flow rate has been at 4 liters per minute, which would require the health unit coordinator to notify the patient's nurse and order the procedure with the specific directions from the respiratory department. pp. 338, 339

NOTES

11. When a patient is "intubated," it means that:
    a. a previously inserted endotracheal tube is removed
    b. an endotracheal or tracheostomy tube has been inserted and placed
    c. he or she is on dialysis
    d. he or she has now been placed on "DNR"

12. Which of the following is used in the treatment of fractures of a cervical vertebra?
    a. Crutchfield's tongs
    b. Steinmann's pins
    c. Buck's traction
    d. Bryant's traction

13. An order for "IPPB 0.5 mL Isuprel c̄ 3 mL NS 20 cm H_2O pressure 10 min tid" means:
    a. respiratory care will perform treatment 10 minutes twice a day
    b. physical therapy will perform treatment 10 minutes three times a day
    c. physical therapy will perform treatment 10 minutes twice a day
    d. respiratory care will perform treatment 10 minutes three times a day

14. In the order "SVN 0.5 cc Albuterol 2.5 cc NS 15 min qid c̄ CPT q 4 hr," CPT means:
    a. chest physiotherapy
    b. continuous positive treatment
    c. chest positive treatment
    d. compressed pressure treatment

15. The order "IS c̄ PEP" is an order for:
    a. incentive spirometry with positive expiratory pressure
    b. inhalation spirometry with prompt expiratory press
    c. incentive spirometry with passive expiratory position
    d. inhalation spirometry with positive expiratory pressure

16. In the doctor's order "MDI c̄ Ventolin ī ī ī puffs qid," MDI is a:
    a. monitored drug inhalation
    b. metered drug inhibitor
    c. metered dose inhaler
    d. monitored dose inhalation

17. A patient with a diagnosis of ESRD has:
    a. renal failure
    b. heart disease
    c. liver failure
    d. pancreatic disease

18. An "A-V shunt creation" is necessary for which of the following procedures?
    a. below-knee amputation
    b. hemodialysis
    c. peritoneal dialysis
    d. open reduction, internal fixation

19. Which of the following crutch training orders would require that the patient not put any weight on the right leg?
    a. crutch training, WBAT rt leg
    b. crutch training, PWB rt leg
    c. crutch training, NWB rt leg
    d. crutch training, TTWB rt leg

20. An order for "PROM to upper extremities" would be a request for the physical therapist to:
    a. administer a heat treatment to the upper extremities
    b. move each joint of the upper extremities to the maximum in each direction
    c. ask the patient to move each joint of the upper extremities to the maximum in each direction
    d. assist the patient in resistive exercises to the upper extremities

☑ *ANSWERS AND RATIONALE*

11. **(b)** Intubation is the insertion and placement of an endotracheal or tracheostomy tube. p. 330

12. **(a)** Crutchfield's tongs are inserted into the skull bones and a traction apparatus is applied to the tongs. This is a treatment for fractured cervical vertebrae. p. 336

13. **(d)** Respiratory care personnel will perform the IPPB (intermittent positive pressure breathing) treatment for 10 minutes tid (three times a day). p. 339

14. **(a)** Chest physiotherapy is a treatment given by respiratory care personnel to loosen and remove secretions from the lung. An SVN (small volume nebulizer) is a treatment similar to IPPB without positive pressure. pp. 331, 340

15. **(a)** "IS c̄ PEP" is an order for incentive spirometry with positive expiratory pressure. p. 341

16. **(c)** Metered dose inhaler (MDI) medication is premeasured in the pharmacy. pp. 331, 341

17. **(a)** ESRD (end-stage renal disease) means that the patient is in renal failure. p. 346

18. **(b)** Hemodialysis would require vascular access. This surgical procedure inserts a cannula into an artery, as well as one into a vein. p. 347

19. **(c)** NWB (non–weight-bearing) rt leg would require that the patient not put any weight on the right leg. pp. 331, 344

WBAT—weight bearing as tolerated
PWB—partial weight bearing
TTWB—toe-touch weight bearing

20. **(b)** "PROM (passive range of motion) to upper extremities" would be a request for the physical therapist to move each joint of the upper extremities to the maximum in each direction. pp. 331, 343

TEST TAKING TIP

Sometimes the option that has the most words is correct. Item writers are aware of this and may try to avoid giving this as a clue.

Miscellaneous Orders

1. A consultation is *usually* requested by the:
   a. patient
   b. attending physician
   c. patient's family
   d. registered nurse

2. Information you should provide when placing a call for a consultation includes the hospital name, your name, patient's name and age, patient's location, person requesting the consultation, patient's diagnosis, and:
   a. patient's identification number
   b. all diagnostic tests that have been ordered
   c. patient's insurance information
   d. names of other doctors consulting

3. The physician may request a patient's old chart from the health record department if the patient has:
   a. previously been treated at the hospital
   b. been in the hospital a long time
   c. gone home on a pass and then returned
   d. always been admitted under the same admitting doctor's name

4. To receive records of diagnostic studies from a patient's stay in a different hospital, a signed consent form must be obtained from:
   a. the previous attending physician
   b. the hospital where the records are stored
   c. the current attending physician
   d. the patient

5. An RN who coordinates the patient's care to improve quality of care while reducing costs is the:
   a. team leader
   b. administrative secretary
   c. case manager
   d. chief financial officer

6. When scheduling a patient for a test or examination performed in a specialized hospital department or outside the hospital, it is important to indicate which of the following on the patient's Kardex form?
   a. length of the test
   b. time of the test
   c. purpose of the test
   d. physician ordering the test

7. Which department would be involved if a patient is admitted with physical injuries and abuse is suspected?
   a. case management
   b. social services
   c. administration
   d. human resources

8. When arranging a temporary absence for a patient, it is necessary to:
   a. complete the discharge procedure
   b. notify social service to go to the patient's home
   c. provide transportation from the hospital
   d. cancel meals during the time of absence

✔ *ANSWERS AND RATIONALE*

1. **(b)** A consultation is usually requested by the attending physician. pp. 350, 351
2. **(c)** The doctor's office will request the patient's insurance information when receiving a call for consultation. p. 351
3. **(a)** The old charts may be requested if the patient has been previously treated at the hospital. p. 352
4. **(d)** Records of a patient's treatment in another hospital are confidential; therefore, obtaining them requires the patient's permission. p. 352
5. **(c)** The case manager is an RN who coordinates the patient's care to improve quality of care while reducing costs. p. 354
6. **(b)** It is important to note the time of the test on the patient's Kardex form. p. 355
7. **(b)** Social services would be called to intervene when a patient is admitted with physical injuries and abuse is suspected. The social worker may call in Adult or Child Protective Services to assess the situation. p. 354
8. **(d)** During temporary absence, all meals must be canceled. p. 355

NOTES

9. When the order for an in-hospital transfer of a patient has been written, it is your responsibility to notify the:
   a. admitting department
   b. business office
   c. clergy
   d. central service department

10. When a patient is designated NINP, it's your responsibility to:
    a. notify the attending physician when he or she arrives on unit or calls
    b. deny having patient on the unit when asked by visitors on unit or by callers
    c. only give status reports about the patient when asked by visitors on unit or callers
    d. order an isolation pack to be placed in the patient's room

11. In the order "Notify hospitalist if systolic blood pressure above 200" the hospitalist is the:
    a. resident on call
    b. emergency room doctor on call
    c. doctor on call for the attending physician
    d. doctor employed by the hospital to care for hospitalized patients

12. If a patient requests no visitors or phone calls, you should notify the:
    a. physician
    b. switchboard
    c. nurse manager
    d. case manager

13. An order for a patient to be discharged with oxygen would require you to notify the:
    a. respiratory department
    b. patient's nurse
    c. case manager
    d. nurse manager

14. An order for which of the following would require the patient or legal guardian to sign a release form?
    a. temporary absence
    b. transfer to another unit
    c. transfer to another room on the same unit
    d. obtaining old charts from health records

15. An order for "DNR" means that the patient:
    a. does not read
    b. will not be resuscitated
    c. is not to be removed from the unit
    d. does not want residents to care for them

☑ ANSWERS AND RATIONALE

9. **(a)** The admitting department must be notified of an in-hospital transfer. p. 356
10. **(b)** NINP (no information, no publication) means the unit denies having the patient when visitors or callers request information. pp. 350, 357
11. **(d)** A hospitalist is a doctor employed by the hospital to care for hospitalized patients. p. 357
12. **(b)** The switchboard must be notified if a patient requests no visitors. p. 357
13. **(c)** An order for discharge with oxygen would require you to notify the case manager, or home care department if applicable. p. 354
14. **(a)** Temporary absence (pass to leave the hospital) would require the patient or legal guardian to sign a release. p. 355
15. **(b)** DNR (do not resuscitate) means that the patient will not receive predetermined life-saving procedures. (This order must be written out by the patient's physician.) pp. 350, 357

TEST TAKING TIP

The number or letter of the correct answer may be the same as several preceding it. When choosing your answer, do not be tempted to vary your answer for this reason.

Health Unit Coordinator Procedures

CHAPTER 19

Admission, Preoperative, and Postoperative Procedures

1. The registration or admitting department is responsible for which of the following tasks when admitting a new patient?
   a. placing a call to the admitting doctor to obtain orders
   b. preparing the facesheet or front sheet
   c. labeling all patient chart forms
   d. assembling the patient chart

2. Which of the following forms serves as a financial agreement between the patient and hospital?
   a. facesheet or front sheet
   b. DRG summary sheet
   c. admission service agreement
   d. advanced directive

3. Which of the following is not included in the information on the identification bracelet?
   a. patient's name
   b. doctor's name
   c. health record number
   d. patient's diagnosis

4. A patient admission form that contains personal demographic information is called a/an:
   a. admission service agreement
   b. facesheet or front sheet
   c. H & P
   d. advanced directive

5. A declaration made by the patient to family, medical staff, and all concerned stating what is to be done in the event that the patient becomes incapacitated is called a/an:
   a. admission service agreement
   b. advanced directive
   c. information sheet
   d. preoperative checklist

6. A patient brought to the hospital by ambulance from an automobile accident would be admitted through the:
   a. outpatient department
   b. admitting department
   c. emergency department
   d. business office

7. The emergency department record of a patient admitted to the hospital is:
   a. sent to the unit with the patient and placed on his or her chart
   b. sent to the health records department
   c. filed with the emergency department records
   d. sent home with the family

8. An observation patient is one who is:
   a. long term and needs to be watched closely
   b. assigned to a bed to receive care for less than 24 hours
   c. a danger to himself or herself as well as to others
   d. terminal

☑ ANSWERS AND RATIONALE

1. **(b)** The admitting department is responsible for preparing the facesheet or front sheet (also may be called the information sheet). pp. 364, 368, 369
2. **(c)** The form that serves as a financial agreement between the patient and the hospital is the admission service agreement form, also may be called the C of A or COA (conditions of admission). pp. 363, 368, 370, 371
3. **(d)** The patient's diagnosis is not included in the information on the patient identification bracelet. p. 368
4. **(b)** The facesheet or front sheet, also called the information sheet, contains patient demographic information. p. 364
5. **(b)** Most states now require that a patient be advised on admission to the hospital of the availability of the advanced directives. pp. 374, 375
6. **(c)** Admissions to the hospital as a result of a medical emergency are processed through the emergency department. pp. 364, 365
7. **(a)** The emergency department record is sent to the nursing unit with the patient and placed on the patient's chart. pp. 365, 366
8. **(b)** An observation patient is assigned to a bed on the nursing unit to receive care for a period of less than 24 hours. This type of patient is also called a short-stay or ambulatory patient. pp. 364, 367

NOTES

9. When the patient arrives on the nursing unit, the first thing the health unit coordinator should do is:
   a. notify the nurse who will be caring for the patient
   b. call the patient's doctor
   c. transcribe the orders
   d. call the admitting department to verify patient information

10. The health unit coordinator may obtain the newly admitted patient's allergy information from the:
   a. patient
   b. conditions of admission sheet
   c. information sheet
   d. nurses' admission record

11. The anesthesiologist's preop orders would include an order for:
   a. the diet
   b. treatments
   c. enemas
   d. name of surgery for consent

12. It is your responsibility to check that the patient's preoperative chart contains a:
   a. recent nurse's note
   b. progress record
   c. history and physical record
   d. vital signs record

13. A patient admitted to the hospital for observation or recovery after surgery for less than 24 hours would be admitted to which of the following units?
   a. emergency unit
   b. medical/surgical unit
   c. medical short-stay unit
   d. intensive care unit

14. Upon arrival, the patient's jewelry may be placed in a valuables envelope and placed in the:
   a. hospital safe
   b. patient's bedside table
   c. unit narcotics cabinet
   d. drawer in the unit nursing station

15. The patient chart form that lists the patient's insurance(s) and nearest relative (next of kin) is the:
   a. progress record
   b. admission service agreement form
   c. facesheet or front sheet
   d. DRG summary sheet

16. A patient is admitted to your unit from the emergency department with written doctor's orders. How would you find out which orders were carried out in the emergency department?
   a. call the emergency department
   b. page the doctor
   c. read the ED record
   d. ask the patient's nurse

17. Power of attorney for health care means that:
   a. the patient's attorney has the right to make medical decisions for the patient if necessary
   b. the hospital attorney will make all decisions for the patient's health care if necessary
   c. the patient's attorney will appoint someone to make health care decisions for the patient if necessary
   d. the patient has appointed another person or persons to make health care decisions for him or her in the event that he or she is unable to do so

18. A "direct admission" means that the patient is admitted:
   a. without a doctor's permission
   b. when he or she prefers to be admitted
   c. not scheduled; from the doctor's office, clinic, or emergency room
   d. when previously scheduled by his or her doctor's office

✔ *ANSWERS AND RATIONALE*

9. **(a)** The nurse caring for the patient should be notified first. p. 376
10. **(d)** The allergy information may be obtained from the nurse's admission record. p. 376
11. **(a)** Preoperative order components from the anesthesiologist are usually diet and medications. p. 380
12. **(c)** It is your responsibility to check the patient's preoperative chart for the history and physical record. p. 381
13. **(c)** The patient would be admitted to the medical short-stay unit (MSSU). The patient may be referred to as an observation patient. pp. 364, 367
14. **(a)** A patient's valuables should always be locked in the hospital safe. pp. 369, 372
15. **(c)** The facesheet or front sheet, also called the information sheet, is the form that would list the patient's insurance(s) and nearest relative (next of kin). pp. 364, 368, 369
16. **(c)** Orders carried out in the emergency department (ED) will be on the ED record. This ED record is sent with the patient and placed in his or her chart. pp. 365, 366
17. **(d)** The patient has appointed another person or persons (called a proxy or agent) to make health care decisions should the patient become incapable of making decisions. p. 375
18. **(c)** A direct admission is not scheduled. The patient is admitted from the doctor's office, clinic, or emergency room. pp. 364, 365

NOTES

19. The surgeon has written an order for a surgery consent to read "right mastectomy." The surgery schedule lists the procedure to be done as "left mastectomy." You should:
   a. notify the nurse and clarify the order with the surgeon
   b. clarify the order with the patient
   c. prepare consent as written by the surgeon and give it to the nurse to have signed
   d. prepare consent as listed on the surgery schedule and give it to the nurse to have signed

20. Which of the following, if missing from the patient's chart, would cause a patient's surgery to be canceled?
   a. signed admission service agreement
   b. advanced directives
   c. nurse's notes from prior admission
   d. doctor's progress notes that were thinned from chart

21. When working on a med/surg unit, you receive a call from the PACU nurse stating that a patient has arrived in the PACU from surgery. You should:
   a. notify the nurse manager
   b. make a note for yourself so you can plan your breaks and be back to transcribe orders
   c. notify the patient's nurse as soon as possible
   d. wait until you receive a call that the patient is returning to his or her room to notify the nurse

22. An elective patient admission is an admission that is:
   a. not planned, but the doctor elects to admit the patient
   b. the result of a car accident or unexpected trauma
   c. not an emergency and can be planned at the patient's and doctor's convenience
   d. dictated by the patient's worsening condition

☑ **ANSWERS AND RATIONALE**

19. **(a)** The nurse should be notified and the order clarified with the surgeon. p. 379
20. **(a)** An unsigned admission service agreement could cause the patient's surgery to be canceled if he or she has received pre-op medication and could not sign the form. pp. 380, 381
21. **(c)** Notify the patient's nurse as soon as possible so the nurse can plan his or her work and be prepared for the patient's return to the unit. p. 391
22. **(c)** An elective patient admission is one that is not an emergency and can be planned at the patient's and doctor's convenience. pp. 364, 365

TEST TAKING TIP

An option may be chosen on an impulse and then on review the option is changed. Avoid this. Studies have shown that the first answer that comes to mind is usually right.

Discharge, Transfer, and Postmortem Procedures

1. The patient's discharge would be initiated when:
   a. the family arrives
   b. the case manager states that everything is arranged for the discharge
   c. the doctor writes the discharge order
   d. the patient states that he or she is ready to leave

2. A patient care conference is held to:
   a. discuss a difficult patient's attitude about his or her care
   b. discuss financial arrangements for a patient's care
   c. make decisions on which doctor will care for patient
   d. plan a patient's care while in the hospital and when discharged

3. Transfer to an ECF differs from a regular discharge in that:
   a. the admitting department must be notified
   b. additional paperwork must be done
   c. the environmental services department is notified
   d. the dietary department is notified

4. Forms that go with a patient to an ECF should be:
   a. sent to the hospital clinic
   b. given to the resident
   c. sent to the doctor's office to be forwarded
   d. placed in a sealed envelope and given to the ambulance driver

5. A patient leaving the hospital AMA:
   a. is leaving without doctor approval
   b. has a disease of interest to the American Medical Association
   c. has asthma-related allergy
   d. has an appointment with medical admissions

6. An autopsy is the same as a:
   a. coroner's case
   b. postmortem
   c. death certification
   d. none of the above

7. A hospitalized patient who dies as a result of stab wounds is considered:
   a. contaminated
   b. a coroner's case
   c. a pathologist's case
   d. a statistic

8. When a patient is transferred to another room in the same hospital, you must:
   a. get a new health record number from admitting
   b. transcribe the transfer orders on a new Kardex
   c. notify the admitting department
   d. cancel treatments and therapies

9. As the discharged patient prepares to leave the nursing unit, you should:
   a. have the patient sign out
   b. obtain hospital personnel to accompany the patient
   c. routinely notify the patient's resident
   d. notify the health records department

☑ *ANSWERS AND RATIONALE*

1. **(c)** The patient's discharge would be initiated when the doctor writes the discharge order. The nurse would then provide the patient with discharge instructions. Transport would need to be arranged to take the patient to the hospital lobby. pp. 396, 397

> It is important to read the doctors' discharge order as the order may read "discharge after chest x-ray" or "discharge after parents receive CPR training." The doctor may leave a prescription in the patient's chart to be given to him or her at time of discharge.

2. **(d)** A patient care conference is held to plan a patient's care while in the hospital and when discharged. p. 396

3. **(b)** Transfer to an ECF differs from a regular discharge in that additional paperwork must be done. p. 401

4. **(d)** Forms are placed in a sealed envelope and sent with the ambulance driver or family member to be given to the nursing staff at the extended care facility (ECF). p. 401

5. **(a)** AMA means against medical advice; therefore, the patient is leaving without doctor approval. pp. 402, 403

6. **(b)** An autopsy is the same as a postmortem. pp. 395, 396, 404

7. **(b)** A coroner's case is one in which the patient's death is due to sudden, violent, or unexplained circumstances. pp. 395, 404

8. **(c)** You must notify the admitting department to get a new room assignment. Often the receiving unit will provide a room number and the health unit coordinator will then notify the admitting department. p. 410

9. **(b)** You should obtain hospital personnel to accompany a patient to the discharge area. p. 397

NOTES

10. In a coroner's case:
    a. family consent must be given for the autopsy
    b. autopsy consent must be obtained prior to the patient's death
    c. the doctor or coroner may obtain autopsy consent
    d. autopsy consent is not required

11. Custodial care means that the patient:
    a. is in legal custody
    b. is taken care of by a nurse custodian
    c. requires around-the-clock nursing
    d. requires care of a nonmedical nature (feeding, bathing, etc.)

12. A patient appears at the nursing station and states that he is leaving the hospital without his doctor's permission. Which of the following would be an appropriate response?
    a. ask the patient to please wait while you notify his nurse
    b. advise the patient that he has a right to leave and allow him to leave
    c. call an orderly to restrain the patient and call the nurse manager
    d. tell the patient he will never get well if he doesn't stay in the hospital

13. When a patient is transferred from ICU to a floor unit or from a floor unit to ICU, the current orders:
    a. remain the same, with additional orders to be written as needed
    b. are no longer valid and new orders are written
    c. are evaluated by the resident, who will discontinue orders as necessary
    d. remain in effect until the attending doctor changes them

14. An order for "organ procurement" indicates that:
    a. the patient is to have surgery that will suspend and secure an organ
    b. the patient's organ is diseased and is nonfunctional
    c. the deceased patient's organ is to be removed
    d. the patent is to receive an organ transplant

15. An order reading "disch with assistance" means that the patient will require:
    a. help getting to his or her car
    b. an ambulance to get home
    c. financial care
    d. home care

16. The health unit coordinator transcribing an order for "DC to home with assistance" would notify:
    a. transport
    b. a CNA
    c. the patient's pastor
    d. the case manager or social worker

17. A patient who dies unexpectedly 2 days after being admitted to the hospital would be:
    a. reported to the local newspaper
    b. turned over to the FBI
    c. a coroner's case
    d. reported to the AMA

☑ **ANSWERS AND RATIONALE**

10. **(d)** An autopsy consent is not required in a coroner's case. p. 404
11. **(d)** Custodial care means that the patient requires care of a nonmedical nature (feeding, bathing, etc.). p. 395
12. **(a)** An appropriate response is to ask the patient to please wait while you notify the nurse. p. 402
13. **(b)** Current orders are no longer valid and new orders are written. p. 411
14. **(c)** Procurement of an organ is the same as harvesting an organ, and means removing an organ from a deceased person who had previously agreed to donate the organ. p. 395
15. **(d)** Discharge with assistance would mean that the patient requires home care (i.e., visiting nurses). p. 401
16. **(d)** The health unit coordinator transcribing an order for "DC to home with assistance" would notify the case manager or social worker. p. 401
17. **(c)** A patient who dies unexpectedly 2 days after being admitted to the hospital would be a coroner's case. p. 404

Recording Vital Signs, Ordering Supplies, Daily Diagnostic Tests, and Filing

1. A doctors' order for routine vital signs requires that the vital signs be checked:
   a. once a day
   b. twice a day
   c. at times defined by hospital policy
   d. three times a day

2. You would record vital signs on which of the following forms?
   a. I & O record
   b. graphic record
   c. DRG sheet
   d. doctor's progress record

3. It is important to record the vital signs in a timely manner so they are available when the:
   a. doctor visits the patient
   b. next set is recorded
   c. patient is discharged
   d. patient is transferred

4. To correct a series of errors on the graphic sheet, you would:
   a. cross through them and write in correct information
   b. have the nurse check the sheet
   c. notify the nurse manager
   d. recopy the graphic sheet, using the correct data

5. Records that come to the nursing unit to be filed on a patient's chart after the patient has been discharged and the chart is no longer on the nursing unit should be:
   a. discarded
   b. mailed to the patient
   c. given to the doctor
   d. forwarded to the health records department

6. The reason daily diagnostic tests should be ordered late in the day for the following day is:
   a. in case the order is canceled by the doctor
   b. so the patient can sleep in
   c. so the nurse may change the order
   d. the health unit coordinator has more time later in the day

7. The reason daily diagnostic tests are performed early in the day is:
   a. the results will be available for the doctors when they make their rounds
   b. the patients will not be interrupted when taking showers or getting bathed
   c. it's not as busy early in the morning because doctors have not made their rounds
   d. it allows more time for preparing the reports

✔ ANSWERS AND RATIONALE

1. **(c)** Times for routine vital signs will vary according to the individual hospital policy. Usually vital signs are taken three times a day. p. 416

2. **(b)** Vital signs are recorded on the graphic sheet. p. 416

> Vital sign graphs are often included in the nursing record, and the nurse is responsible for recording his or her patient's vital signs.

3. **(a)** Recorded vital signs should be available for the doctors when they visit their patients. p. 416

4. **(d)** To correct a series of errors on the graphic sheet, the entire sheet needs to be recopied using the correct data. The original graphic sheet would be placed in the chart with one line drawn across the entire sheet and a notation that it has been recopied, with the date, time, and name of the person who recopied it. p. 416

5. **(d)** The records need to be forwarded to the health records department, where they will be added to the patient's chart. p. 421

6. **(a)** Daily diagnostic tests should be ordered late in the day for the following day in case they are canceled. p. 422

7. **(a)** Daily diagnostic tests are performed early in the day so the results will be available for the doctors when they make their rounds. p. 422

NOTES

8. Daily diagnostic tests are performed every day until:
   a. the test results are within the normal range
   b. a doctor's order discontinues the test
   c. a nurse cancels the order
   d. the testing department decides the patient no longer needs the test

9. When filing records or reports on a patient's chart, it is important to:
   a. note whether the record or report is signed
   b. check the patient name on the chart with the patient name on the record or report
   c. check the chart to see whether the test or procedure was ordered
   d. show each record or report to the patient's nurse before filing

10. To order a flashlight for the nursing unit, you would contact which of the following departments?
    a. central service
    b. purchasing
    c. environmental services
    d. pharmacy

11. Alcohol sponges are obtained from which of the following departments?
    a. environmental services
    b. pharmacy
    c. central service
    d. laboratory

12. Nourishments for the nursing unit are ordered from which of the following?
    a. central service
    b. dietary
    c. environmental service
    d. cafeteria

13. The cost of linen supplies is usually absorbed in the:
    a. nursing unit budget
    b. charge for the patient's room
    c. charging of individual items to the patient
    d. hospital administration

☑ *ANSWERS AND RATIONALE*

8. **(b)** Daily diagnostic tests are ordered each day until discontinued by a doctor's order. p. 422

9. **(b)** Check the patient name on the chart with the patient name on the record or report. pp. 417, 421

10. **(b)** A flashlight is ordered from the purchasing department. p. 422

11. **(c)** Alcohol sponges are obtained from the central service department. p. 422

12. **(b)** Nourishments are obtained from the dietary department. p. 424

13. **(b)** The cost of the linens is usually absorbed in the charge for the patient's room. p. 424

Reports, Infection Control, Emergencies, and Special Services

1. The discovery of a fire on a unit requires the health unit coordinator to immediately notify the:
   a. hospital fire marshal
   b. hospital telephone operator
   c. security
   d. fire department

2. Flowers may be restricted on which two of the following units?
   1. telemetry unit   a. 1 & 3
   2. oncology unit   b. 2 & 4
   3. respiratory unit   c. 3 & 4
   4. ICU   d. 4 & 5
   5. neurology unit

3. An incident report is initiated if a:
   a. patient refuses a pain medication
   b. nurse is late for work
   c. medication is omitted
   d. therapy is canceled

4. A copy of the incident report would go to which of the following?
   a. the patient
   b. the nurse manager
   c. the doctor
   d. the health records department

5. Reverse isolation is used when a patient:
   a. has been exposed to a contagious disease
   b. has a contagious disease
   c. is susceptible to infection
   d. has a hospital-acquired infection

6. Which of the following is a common hospital-acquired infection?
   a. pneumonitis
   b. pseudomonas
   c. mononucleosis
   d. coccidioidomycosis

7. Pathogens are not usually transmitted by:
   a. air
   b. personal contact
   c. inanimate objects
   d. body excretion

8. When a code arrest is called for a patient, it means:
   a. his or her heart or breathing has stopped
   b. his or her insurance has been canceled
   c. he or she is under arrest
   d. there is a fire within the hospital

9. When a patient suffers a code arrest, you should first call the:
   a. attending doctor
   b. resident
   c. nurse manager
   d. hospital telephone operator

10. When a patient suffers a code arrest, your main responsibility is to:
    a. stay at the desk
    b. perform CPR
    c. call each department to send someone to the floor
    d. go to ICU and arrange for a bed

✔ ANSWERS AND RATIONALE

1. **(b)** The hospital telephone operator would announce the code, alerting all hospital personnel. p. 434

2. **(c)** The respiratory unit and the ICU may restrict flowers. The health unit coordinator would ask the family to take the flowers home. p. 435

3. **(c)** Incident reports are required for accidents, thefts, errors of omission, or errors in administration of patient medication or treatments. p. 428

4. **(b)** A copy of the incident report would go to the nurse manager. Incident reports are never a part of the patient's permanent record. p. 428

5. **(c)** Reverse isolation is a precautionary measure that is practiced to prevent a patient with impaired or low resistance to disease from being infected. p. 432

6. **(b)** The three organisms usually responsible for hospital-acquired infections are *Streptococcus, Staphylococcus,* and *Pseudomonas.* p. 433

7. **(c)** Pathogens are usually not transmitted by inanimate objects. Pathogens may be transmitted by air, personal contact, and body excretions. p. 430

8. **(a)** A code arrest means that the patient's heart or breathing has stopped. pp. 427, 434

9. **(d)** The hospital telephone operator is notified immediately to announce the code. The code team will respond to the code when it is announced by the operator. pp. 434, 435

10. **(a)** Your responsibilities during a code arrest are performed from the desk area. (Your responsibilities include directing the code team to the room, ordering tests and procedures, and placing necessary phone calls.) p. 435

NOTES

11. In the event of a hospital fire:
    a. the staff is notified by overhead announcement of code name and/or number
    b. the staff is notified by a fireman who goes to affected units
    c. transport personnel go from unit to unit
    d. the health unit coordinator closest to the fire calls each unit in the hospital

12. An example of a situation in which a hospital would institute a disaster procedure is:
    a. 20% of the staff calling in sick
    b. a train wreck
    c. a car accident with two or more injuries
    d. a trauma patient brought in by helicopter

13. Standard precautions are used:
    a. to make it easier for employees to transfer to any unit in the hospital
    b. only when patients have a communicable disease
    c. in critical care units
    d. to create a barrier between the health care worker and the patient's body fluids

14. AIDS stands for:
    a. acquired immunodeficiency syndrome
    b. activated immunovirus disease symptoms
    c. activated immunodeficiency syndrome
    d. acquired immuno disease syndrome

15. The following patient condition would not be entered into the computer when ordering a test:
    a. RSV
    b. HBV
    c. PID
    d. AIDS

16. A patient would be placed in AFB isolation to prevent transmission of:
    a. AIDS
    b. RSV
    c. TB
    d. HBV

17. A condition also transmitted by body fluids that is more contagious than AIDS is:
    a. HBV
    b. RA
    c. PID
    d. URI

18. A laboratory phlebotomist informs you that he or she performed a lab test on the wrong patient. After notifying the appropriate nurses and doctors, you would:
    a. call the lab supervisor
    b. call risk management
    c. prepare an incident report
    d. notify the involved patient's families

☑ ANSWERS AND RATIONALE

11. **(a)** A code name and/or number (e.g., code 1000) is announced by the hospital telephone operator to avoid using the term *fire*. p. 434

12. **(b)** Disasters may occur during a flood, fire, bombing, or accident such as a train wreck or plane crash. p. 434

13. **(d)** Standard precautions are used to create a barrier between the health care worker and the patient's body fluids. pp. 428, 431

14. **(a)** AIDS stands for acquired immunodeficiency syndrome. pp. 428, 432

15. **(d)** AIDS (acquired immunodeficiency syndrome) would not be entered into the computer. p. 433

Laws regarding AIDS and confidentiality vary from state to state, as do laws regarding disclosure of HIV-positive persons. When in doubt, do not disclose information. In most health care facilities, guidelines such as not entering the AIDS diagnosis on the computer have been established to assist the health care worker.

16. **(c)** A patient would be placed in isolation to prevent transmission of TB (tuberculosis). AFB stands for acid-fast bacilli, which cause tuberculosis. p. 432

AIDS—acquired immunodeficiency syndrome
HBV—hepatitis B virus
RSV—respiratory syncytial virus

17. **(a)** HBV (hepatitis B virus) is also transmitted by body fluids and is more contagious than AIDS. p. 433

PID—pelvic inflammatory disease
RA—rheumatoid arthritis
URI—upper respiratory infection

18. **(c)** Documentation of all incidents is important in the case of a lawsuit arising from them. Incidents are studied and trends derived in an attempt to prevent similar incidents from happening in the future. pp. 428–430

SECTION

5

Introduction to Anatomic Structures, Medical Terms, and Illnesses

23

Medical Terminology, Basic Human Structure, Diseases, and Disorders

Many questions in this chapter are not in the format that is used in the certification test but will be helpful in your basic understanding of the material.

UNIT 2: Body Structure and Skin

1. The basic unit of all living things is the:
   a. cell
   b. cytoplasm
   c. heart
   d. skin

2. The three main parts of a cell are:
   a. tissue, cytoplasm, cell membrane
   b. tissue, organ, system
   c. protoplasm, cell membrane, nucleus
   d. cell membrane, cytoplasm, nucleus

3. Tissue is made up of:
   a. similar cells
   b. different cells
   c. similar organs
   d. different organs

4. Which of the following is a body organ?
   a. cell
   b. tissue
   c. ureter
   d. nucleus

5. The spleen is located in which of the following cavities?
   a. cranial
   b. thoracic
   c. abdominal
   d. pelvic

6. A doctor's order that includes a chest x-ray to be taken from an anterior view would mean that the x-ray machine would be positioned at the patient's:
   a. back
   b. front
   c. rt side
   d. lt side

7. A doctor's order that includes the term inferior is referring to:
   a. below
   b. above
   c. in front of
   d. in back of

8. A doctor's order for a side view x-ray would be which of the following?
   a. lateral
   b. medial
   c. anterior
   d. posterior

☑ ANSWERS AND RATIONALE

1. **(a)** The basic unit of all life is the cell. p. 447
2. **(d)** The three main parts of a cell are the cell membrane, cytoplasm, and nucleus. p. 448
3. **(a)** Tissue is made up of similar cells. p. 448
4. **(c)** The ureter, a tube that leads from each kidney to the bladder, is a body organ. p. 448
5. **(c)** The spleen is located in the abdominal cavity. p. 449
6. **(b)** Anterior means in front of (or ventral). p. 450
7. **(a)** Inferior means below (or caudal). p. 450
8. **(a)** Lateral means pertaining to the side. p. 450

TEST-TAKING TIP

When taking the test, take time to read the test-taking directions, then follow them carefully. Failure to do so may result in your correct answer being scored by the machine as a wrong answer. If, for example, your pencil mark is not in the exact required space, the machine may read it as an incorrect answer. Check that each question number matches the answer number. Do not hesitate to ask questions if you do not know how to proceed.

9. Which of the following is a function of the skin?
   a. protection from pathogenic microorganisms
   b. regulation of extracellular materials
   c. transportation of nutrients and oxygen to cells
   d. exchange of gases

10. The outer layer of the skin is called:
    a. epidermis
    b. dermis
    c. subcutaneous
    d. porous

11. Which of the following is the death of body tissue caused by a lack of blood supply to an area of the body?
    a. abscess
    b. cancer
    c. gangrene
    d. laceration

12. A term used in the doctor's progress notes that means disease producing is:
    a. pathology
    b. carcinogenic
    c. pathogenic
    d. carcinoma

13. A term used in the patient's H&P that means resembling hair is:
    a. cytoid
    b. trichoid
    c. dermatoid
    d. sternoid

14. Which of the following terms used in the patient's pathology report would indicate that the tumor removed consisted of connective tissue?
    a. lipoma
    b. sarcoma
    c. myoma
    d. epithelioma

15. A specimen collected by the doctor for "study of cells" would be sent to:
    a. dermatology
    b. histology
    c. cytology
    d. pathology

16. A term frequently seen in the doctor's progress notes or in the patient's H&P when referring to internal organs is:
    a. epithelial
    b. visceral
    c. dermal
    d. abdominal

> **UNIT 3: The Musculoskeletal System**

17. A patient admitted to the hospital with a broken upper jaw has a fracture of the:
    a. maxilla
    b. mandible
    c. malleus
    d. metacarpal

18. A doctor's order for an x-ray of the pelvic bones would include which of the following?
    a. lumbar, sacrum, coccyx
    b. ilium, ischium, pubis
    c. ischium, ilium, sacrum
    d. pubis, ischium, ileum

19. Which of the following bones form the upper sides of the cranium?
    a. temporal
    b. ethmoid
    c. sphenoid
    d. parietal

20. A CT of the first seven vertebrae would be a CT of which vertebrae?
    a. cervical
    b. thoracic
    c. lumbar
    d. sacral

21. An x-ray of the wrist would include which of these bones?
    a. tarsals
    b. metatarsals
    c. carpals
    d. metacarpals

22. A patient admitted with a fracture of the lower arm, thumb side, would have a fractured:
    a. ulna
    b. humerus
    c. radius
    d. tibia

☑ *ANSWERS AND RATIONALE*

9. **(a)** Protection from pathogenic microorganisms is a function of the integumentary system. p. 450

10. **(a)** The epidermis, which contains no blood vessels, is the outer layer of the skin. The dermis is often referred to as the true skin. p. 450

11. **(c)** Gangrene is the death of body tissue caused by a lack of blood supply to an area of the body. p. 452

12. **(c)** Pathogenic means disease producing. p. 459

13. **(b)** Trichoid means resembling hair. p. 459

14. **(b)** Sarcoma is a tumor composed of connective tissue. p. 459

15. **(c)** Cytology means study of cells. p. 459

16. **(b)** Visceral means internal organs. p. 459

17. **(a)** Maxilla is the name for the upper jaw bone. p. 464

18. **(b)** The pelvic bones are composed of the ilium, ischium, and pubis. p. 465. The ileum is a portion of the small intestine. p. 521.

19. **(d)** The parietal bones form the upper sides of the cranium. p. 464

20. **(a)** The cervical vertebrae form the neck. p. 464

21. **(c)** The carpals form the wrist. p. 465

22. **(c)** The radius is the lower arm bone, thumb side. p. 465

NOTES

23. Muscles are attached to bone by:
    a. ligaments
    b. tendons
    c. nerves
    d. joints

24. Which of the following procedures may be performed for treatment of a herniated nucleus pulposus?
    a. arthroplasty
    b. laminectomy
    c. laparotomy
    d. chondrectomy

25. A fracture with a broken bone and an open wound in the skin is called:
    a. simple
    b. compound
    c. greenstick
    d. closed

26. Tough bands of tissue that connect one bone to another bone at a joint are called:
    a. periosteum
    b. ligament
    c. tendon
    d. muscle

27. A term used in a doctor's order referring to the thigh bone would be:
    a. tibial
    b. humeral
    c. femoral
    d. femeral

28. The doctor's surgical report referring to below the ribs would contain the term:
    a. subscapular
    b. suprascapular
    c. subcostal
    d. sublingual

29. A consent for surgical incision into the collar bone would be a consent for a:
    a. chondrectomy
    b. costectomy
    c. craniotomy
    d. clavicotomy

30. A patient has a crippling disease of the muscle. The admitting diagnosis is:
    a. muscular dystrophy
    b. muscular atrophy
    c. myocardial infarction
    d. multiple sclerosis

31. In the progress notes, the doctor would use which of the following terms to indicate "between the vertebrae"?
    a. intravertebral
    b. vertebrocostal
    c. vertebrectomy
    d. intervertebral

32. The doctor would use which instrument to visualize a joint?
    a. arthrogram
    b. arthroscope
    c. arthroscopy
    d. arthrotomy

33. The doctor would perform which of the following to obtain bone marrow for study?
    a. sternoclavicular
    b. sternocostal
    c. sternal puncture
    d. sternotomy

34. The process of recording electrical activity of muscle is:
    a. electromyograph
    b. electromyography
    c. electromyogram
    d. electrocardiography

35. The patient's H&P indicates that the patient has an inflammation of the cartilage or:
    a. chondritis
    b. arthritis
    c. arthrosis
    d. chondrogenic

36. Paget's disease is a disease of the:
    a. pancreas
    b. liver
    c. bone
    d. lung

37. Prevention of osteoporosis would include which of the following supplements?
    a. potassium
    b. vitamin C
    c. calcium
    d. magnesium

☑ ANSWERS AND RATIONALE

23. **(b)** Muscles are attached to bone by tendons. p. 466
24. **(b)** A laminectomy, which is the surgical removal of a portion of the vertebra, may be performed as a treatment for herniated nucleus pulposus, also called a herniated or slipped disc. p. 467
25. **(b)** An open compound fracture is a broken bone and an open wound. p. 468
26. **(b)** Ligaments connect bones at a joint. p. 466
27. **(c)** Femoral means pertaining to the thigh bone. p. 475
28. **(c)** Subcostal means pertaining to below the ribs. p. 475
29. **(d)** Clavicotomy means surgical incision into the collar bone. p. 475
30. **(a)** Muscular dystrophy is a crippling disease of the muscle. p. 475
31. **(d)** Intervertebral means pertaining to between the vertebrae. *Inter* means between, whereas *intra* means within. p. 475
32. **(b)** An arthroscope is the instrument used to visualize a joint. *Scope* means instrument, whereas *scopy* means the examination. p. 476
33. **(c)** Sternal puncture is performed to obtain bone marrow. p. 476
34. **(b)** Electromyography is the process of recording the electrical activity of muscle. *Graph* means instrument used to record, whereas *gram* means record. p. 476
35. **(a)** Chondritis means inflammation of the cartilage. p. 475
36. **(c)** Paget's disease is a condition that affects the bone. p. 468
37. **(c)** Calcium supplements, exercise, hormone replacement therapy (if appropriate), and correct posture are recommended as preventative measures. p. 467

NOTES

UNIT 4: The Nervous System

38. The brain is divided into three main parts, consisting of the:
    a. cerebrum, spinal cord, brain stem
    b. cerebrum, cerebellum, brain stem
    c. brain stem, nerves, cerebellum
    d. cerebrosis, cerebellum, brain stem

39. Which of the following transmits nerve impulses from the brain to the spinal cord?
    a. ventricles
    b. dura mater
    c. sensory neurons
    d. motor neurons

40. The ventricles produce which of the following?
    a. nerve impulses
    b. red blood cells
    c. cerebrospinal fluid
    d. electrical stimuli

41. Following a CVA, the patient is experiencing loss of memory and motor function. This is probably caused by tissue damage to the:
    a. cerebellum
    b. cerebrum
    c. brain stem
    d. spinal cord

42. The spinal cord extends from the brain to:
    a. between the first and second lumbar vertebrae
    b. below the fourth lumbar vertebra
    c. the sacrum
    d. between the 10th and 11th thoracic vertebrae

43. A patient having an injury to the spinal cord may experience a loss of:
    a. vision
    b. hearing
    c. memory
    d. muscle function

44. The meninges are made up of which of the following layers?
    a. dura mater, arachnoid, pia mater
    b. dura mater, ventricles, pia mater
    c. dura mater, spinal cord, pia mater
    d. dura mater, subarachnoid space, pia mater

45. A patient who complains of loss of balance may have a disease or condition of the:
    a. brain stem
    b. cerebellum
    c. cerebrum
    d. aqueous humor

46. Impaired blood supply to parts of the brain is called a stroke or:
    a. cerebral palsy
    b. coronary vascular accident
    c. coronary thrombosis
    d. cerebrovascular accident

47. Which of the following is considered a warning sign for stroke and is characterized by recurrent episodes of decreased neurological function?
    a. CVA
    b. CHF
    c. TIA
    d. TUR

48. Which of the following diseases is characterized by loss of memory, restlessness, and inability to carry out purposeful movement?
    a. Parkinson's disease
    b. Alzheimer's disease
    c. Cushing's disease
    d. Addison's disease

49. Following a spinal cord injury, a patient may have paralysis of her legs, or:
    a. paraplegia
    b. quadriplegia
    c. hemiplegia
    d. ophthalmoplegia

50. What is the correct spelling of the medical term meaning suturing of a nerve?
    a. neurorrhaphy   3R 2h
    b. neurorrhapy
    c. neurorraphy
    d. neurorhaphy

51. A patient diagnosed as having multiple sclerosis would seek treatment from a/an:
    a. urologist
    b. orthopedist
    c. neurologist
    d. psychiatrist

☑ ANSWERS AND RATIONALE

38. **(b)** The brain consists of the cerebrum, cerebellum, and brain stem. p. 482

39. **(d)** Motor neurons carry impulses away from the brain, whereas sensory neurons transmit impulses to the brain. p. 482

40. **(c)** The ventricles produce cerebrospinal fluid, which surrounds the brain and spinal cord and acts as a cushion. p. 482

41. **(b)** The cerebrum contains sensory, motor, sight, and hearing centers. Memory, intellect, judgment, and emotional reactions also take place in the cerebrum. p. 482

42. **(a)** The spinal cord extends to between the first and second lumbar vertebrae. p. 482

43. **(d)** Injury to the spinal cord may interfere with the transmitting of motor impulses, resulting in loss of muscle function. p. 482

44. **(a)** Dura mater, arachnoid, and pia mater make up the meninges. p. 482

45. **(b)** Balance is a function of the cerebellum. p. 482

46. **(d)** A cerebrovascular accident (CVA) is a result of impaired blood supply to parts of the brain. p. 482

47. **(c)** A TIA (transient ischemic attack) is characterized by double vision, slurred speech, weakness in the legs, and dizziness, lasting from seconds to 24 hours and then clearing. pp. 482, 483

48. **(b)** Symptoms of Alzheimer's disease, which usually begins in mid-life and is progressive, include memory loss, restlessness, and inability to carry out purposeful movement. p. 483

49. **(a)** Paraplegia is the paralysis of the legs and sometimes the lower part of the body, and is usually the result of a spinal cord injury. p. 487

50. **(a)** Neurorrhaphy is the correct spelling. Note that the suffix *orrhaphy*, which means to suture, has two r's and two h's. p. 487

51. **(c)** A patient with multiple sclerosis, a degenerative disease involving the brain and spinal cord, would seek treatment from a neurologist, one who treats diseases of the nervous system. p. 487

NOTES

52. A viral disease that attacks the gray matter of the spinal cord is:
    a. poliomyelitis
    b. epilepsy
    c. encephalitis
    d. cerebellitis

53. Which of the following terms would be printed on a surgical schedule?
    a. neuroma
    b. neuropathy
    c. neuralgia
    d. neuroplasty

54. A patient is admitted with inflammation of the brain. The admitting diagnosis would be:
    a. encephalitis
    b. meningitis
    c. poliomyelitis
    d. cerebellitis

55. Which of the following conditions involve the herniation of the spinal cord and meninges?
    a. encephalocele
    b. meningomyelocele
    c. cerebral palsy
    d. meningomyelorrhea

56. A procedure that may be ordered by the doctor to determine brain death is a/an:
    a. electroencephalogram
    b. pneumoencephalogram
    c. echoencephalogram
    d. arthrogram

57. The procedure used to obtain CSF is a/an:
    a. pelvic examination
    b. lumbar puncture
    c. myringotomy
    d. abdominocentesis

58. One who studies the mind is a:
    a. neurologist
    b. psychologist
    c. psychiatrist
    d. physiatrist

59. Which of the following terms refers to a mental disorder?
    a. neurosis
    b. psychosis
    c. psychosomatic
    d. neurotic

60. A condition recognized by symptoms including muscle rigidity, tremors, and a shifting gait is:
    a. Alzheimer's disease
    b. Parkinson's disease
    c. Graves' disease
    d. diabetes mellitus

61. Epilepsy is a disease of the:
    a. blood
    b. central nervous system
    c. bone
    d. peripheral nervous system

62. An appropriate action to take when caring for a patient having an epileptic seizure would be to:
    a. place a pillow under the patient's head if possible
    b. remove any furniture or other objects that the patient may strike
    c. call for help
    d. all of the above

UNIT 5: The Eye and the Ear

63. The transparent membrane that lines the upper and lower eyelid and the anterior portion of the eye is called the:
    a. choroid
    b. conjunctiva
    c. sclera
    d. cornea

64. The middle layer of the eye is called the:
    a. choroid
    b. retina
    c. sclera
    d. cornea

65. The anterior middle portion of the choroid is made up of the:
    a. sclera and cornea
    b. pupil and ciliary muscle
    c. iris and pupil
    d. iris and ciliary muscle

66. The cornea is known as the:
    a. white of the eye
    b. transparent part of the sclera
    c. regulator of the shape of the eye
    d. protector of the eye from harmful bacteria

☑ ANSWERS AND RATIONALE

52. **(a)** Poliomyelitis is a viral disease that attacks the gray matter of the spinal cord. p. 488

53. **(d)** Neuroplasty is a surgical term; therefore, it would appear on the surgery schedule. p. 487

54. **(a)** Encephalitis means inflammation of the brain. Cerebellitis means *inflammation of the cerebellum* only and not the whole brain. p. 487

55. **(b)** Meningomyelocele means herniation of the spinal cord and meninges. p. 488

56. **(a)** An electroencephalogram (EEG) is a tracing or recording of the electrical impulses of the brain. p. 488

57. **(b)** A lumbar puncture, or spinal tap, is used to obtain cerebral spinal fluid (CSF). p. 488

58. **(b)** A psychologist is one who studies the mind, whereas a psychiatrist is a physician who deals with the study, treatment, and prevention of mental illness. p. 492

59. **(b)** Psychosis is a mental disorder. p. 492

60. **(b)** Parkinson's disease, also called shaking palsy, is one of the most crippling diseases in the United States. p. 483

    Alzheimer's disease is characterized by confusion, loss of memory, restlessness, hallucinations, and the inability to carry out purposeful movement. p. 483

    Graves' disease is a form of hyperthyroidism. pp. 569, 571

    Diabetes mellitus is a disease that results in the inability of the body to store and use carbohydrates in the usual manner. pp. 569, 571

61. **(b)** Epilepsy is a disease of the central nervous system. p. 483

62. **(d)** In addition to those actions noted in question, a patient having an epileptic seizure should not have his or her movements restrained. p. 483

63. **(b)** The conjunctiva lines the eye and serves to protect it from harmful bacteria. p. 493

64. **(a)** The middle layer of the eye is the choroid, which contains blood vessels that supply nutrients to the eye. p. 494

65. **(d)** The iris and ciliary muscle make up the anterior middle portion of the choroid. The iris, the colored portion of the eye, has an opening in the center called the pupil. p. 494

66. **(b)** The cornea is the transparent part of the sclera that lies over the iris and allows light rays to enter. p. 493

NOTES

67. The dilation and contraction of the pupil of the eye are regulated by the muscles of the:
   a. iris
   b. pupil
   c. choroid
   d. sclera

68. The eye receives light rays that are focused on the:
   a. choroid
   b. cornea
   c. lens
   d. retina

69. The large posterior space behind the lens is filled with a jellylike substance called the:
   a. aqueous humor
   b. vitreous humor
   c. choroid
   d. ciliary body

70. What are the three layers of the eye?
   a. pupil, lens, iris
   b. conjunctiva, cornea, optic nerve
   c. sclera, choroid, retina
   d. vitreous humor, aqueous humor, dry humor

71. Phacoemulsification is a surgical procedure used to treat:
   a. glaucoma
   b. strabismus
   c. retinal detachment
   d. cataracts

72. Maintaining equilibrium is a function of the:
   a. cerebrum
   b. brain stem
   c. ear
   d. thymus gland

73. The small snail-shaped structure next to the oval window in the inner ear is the:
   a. semicircular canals
   b. cochlea
   c. auditory nerve
   d. incus

74. The eustachian tube leads from the middle ear to the:
   a. pharynx
   b. outer ear
   c. inner ear
   d. larynx

75. The ossicles consist of the:
   a. malleus, incus, and stapes
   b. malleus, stapes, and cochlea
   c. incus, stapes, and cochlea
   d. incus, stapes, and tympanic membrane

76. A patient scheduled for a blepharoplasty would be having surgical repair of the:
   a. lip
   b. eyelid
   c. iris
   d. eyebrow

77. The word root for cornea is:
   a. irid/o
   b. kerat/o
   c. retin/o
   d. blephar/o

78. Surgery for removal of a clouded lens would be listed on the surgery schedule as a/an:
   a. ophthalmectomy
   b. cataract extraction
   c. enucleation
   d. sclerotomy

79. Which of the following conditions is the result of a weakness in the eye muscle?
   a. glaucoma
   b. strabismus
   c. retinal detachment
   d. keratocele

80. The correct spelling of the term that means discharge from the ear is:
   a. otorrhea
   b. otorhea
   c. otorrea
   d. otarrhea

81. Which of the following instruments is kept on the nursing unit?
   a. proctoscope
   b. bronchoscope
   c. ophthalmoscope
   d. arthroscope

82. A child suffering from otitis media would complain of pain in the:
   a. ear
   b. nose
   c. throat
   d. eye

☑ *ANSWERS AND RATIONALE*

67. **(a)** The muscles of the iris regulate the dilation and contraction of the pupil. p. 494

68. **(d)** The light rays received by the eye are focused on the retina. pp. 493, 494

69. **(b)** The substance that fills the large posterior space behind the lens is called vitreous humor. Its function is to maintain the shape of the eyeball and to assist in bending light rays. p. 495

70. **(c)** The three layers of the eye are the sclera, choroid, and retina. p. 493

71. **(d)** Phacoemulsification, the use of ultrasonic vibrations to break the lens into pieces that are then aspirated, is used to treat cataracts. p. 495

72. **(c)** Maintaining equilibrium and hearing are the two functions of the ear. p. 495

73. **(b)** The cochlea, shaped like a snail, is the structure next to the oval window in the ear. p. 495

74. **(a)** The eustachian tube, which leads from the middle ear to the pharynx, equalizes pressure on both sides of the tympanic membrane. p. 495

75. **(a)** The ossicles are made up of the malleus, incus, and stapes. p. 495

76. **(b)** Blepharoplasty is the surgical repair of the eyelid. p. 500

77. **(b)** The word root for cornea is *kerat/o*. p. 499

78. **(b)** Cataract extraction is surgery to remove a clouded lens. p. 500

79. **(b)** Strabismus, or crossed eyes, is a condition resulting from weakness of the eye muscle. p. 500

80. **(a)** Otorrhea is the correct spelling. *Ot/o* is the combining form for *ear. Orrhea* is from the grouping of *-rrh* suffixes that also includes *-rrhagia* and *-rrhaphy*. p. 500

81. **(c)** The ophthalmoscope is kept on the nursing unit. The other instruments listed are used for more complex examination and therefore are stored in special examining rooms. p. 500

82. **(a)** Otitis media is the inflammation of the middle ear; therefore, the child would experience pain in the middle ear. p. 500

NOTES

83. The medical term for pinkeye is:
    a. conjunctivitis
    b. otitis media
    c. sclerokeratitis
    d. scleritis

84. A middle ear infection is causing pressure on the eardrum. An incision into the eardrum to release the pressure and to allow for drainage is called a:
    a. blepharotomy
    b. sclerotomy
    c. myringotomy
    d. stapedectomy

85. Rods and cones are sets of nerve cells that transmit impulses to the:
    a. optic nerve
    b. retina
    c. auditory canal
    d. auditory nerve

86. A name given to a condition of ringing, buzzing, or roaring noises in the ears is:
    a. tympanitis
    b. myringitis
    c. otitis media
    d. tinnitus

> ### UNIT 6: The Circulatory System

87. The partition dividing the heart into the right and left sides is called the:
    a. septum
    b. bicuspid valve
    c. tricuspid valve
    d. mitral valve

88. Which of the following body systems is responsible for carrying food, oxygen, waste, and other materials needed for cell function?
    a. digestive
    b. circulatory
    c. endocrine
    d. respiratory

89. Which of the following carries oxygenated blood?
    a. inferior vena cava
    b. aorta
    c. superior vena cava
    d. pulmonary artery

90. Blood returns to the right atrium of the heart through which of the following?
    a. aorta
    b. pulmonary vein
    c. superior vena cava
    d. pulmonary artery

91. The exchange of substances between the blood and body cells takes place while the blood is in the:
    a. venules
    b. arterioles
    c. lungs
    d. capillaries

92. The fluid portion of the blood is called:
    a. platelets
    b. plasma
    c. leukocytes
    d. erythrocytes

93. A sternal puncture is performed by doctors to determine:
    a. bone density
    b. erythrocyte production
    c. bone marrow capacity
    d. leukocyte production

94. To diagnose appendicitis, the doctor may order which of the following laboratory tests to determine the presence of infection in the body?
    a. white blood cell count
    b. red blood cell count
    c. platelet count
    d. hemoglobin

95. The prime function of platelets is to:
    a. aid in clotting blood
    b. carry oxygen
    c. fight pathogenic microorganisms
    d. release histamines

96. Which of the following structures pumps blood through the pulmonary artery?
    a. right atrium
    b. left ventricle
    c. right ventricle
    d. left atrium

97. The bicuspid valve is located between the:
    a. left atrium and left ventricle
    b. right atrium and right ventricle
    c. right ventricle and pulmonary artery
    d. left ventricle and aorta

☑ ANSWERS AND RATIONALE

83. **(a)** Conjunctivitis is the medical term for pinkeye. p. 500

84. **(c)** Myringotomy means incision into the tympanic membrane or eardrum. p. 500

85. **(a)** Rods and cones send impulses to the optic nerve. p. 494

86. **(d)** Tinnitus is a condition that causes a ringing, buzzing, or roaring noise in the ears. pp. 495, 496

87. **(a)** The septum divides the heart into the right and left sides. p. 504

88. **(b)** The heart pumps the blood, which carries food, oxygen, waste, and other materials through the blood vessels to the lungs and other body cells. p. 504

89. **(b)** The aorta, the largest artery in the body, carries oxygenated blood away from the left ventricle of the heart. p. 504

90. **(c)** The superior and inferior venae cavae are large veins through which the blood returns to the atrium from the body. p. 504

91. **(d)** While the blood is in the capillaries (microscopic, thin-walled blood vessels), the exchange of nutrients, oxygen, and carbon dioxide between the blood and body cells takes place. p. 504

92. **(b)** Plasma is the fluid portion of the blood. It is approximately 90% water. Blood cells are suspended in the plasma. p. 507

93. **(b)** Erythrocytes are produced by the red bone marrow found in the flat bones of the body, such as the sternum. A sternal puncture is performed to obtain a red bone marrow specimen in order to study its ability to produce erythrocytes. p. 507

94. **(a)** White blood cells, or leukocytes, fight against disease-causing bacteria. An elevated white blood cell count may indicate infection in the body. p. 507

95. **(a)** The prime function of platelets is to aid in clotting the blood. p. 507

96. **(c)** The right ventricle pumps blood through the pulmonary arteries, whereas the left ventricle pumps blood through the aorta to the body parts. p. 507

97. **(a)** The bicuspid valve separates the left atrium from the left ventricle. The tricuspid valve separates the right atrium from the right ventricle. p. 504

NOTES

98. As the blood is circulating through the heart, it travels from the pulmonary vein to the:
    a. right atrium
    b. left ventricle
    c. right ventricle
    d. left atrium

99. A function of the spleen is to:
    a. store blood for emergency use
    b. produce platelets
    c. produce insulin
    d. secrete bile

100. Buildup of plaque on the arterial walls that leads to blockage is called:
    a. arteriosclerosis
    b. aneurysm
    c. atherosclerosis
    d. arteriostenosis

101. A patient scheduled for the surgical removal of enlarged veins in the rectal area will have an order for a/an:
    a. herniorrhaphy
    b. hemorrhoidectomy
    c. hemorroidectomy
    d. angiorrhaphy

102. Which of the following conditions is commonly referred to as a heart attack?
    a. coronary thrombosis
    b. pulmonary thrombosis
    c. coronary aneurysm
    d. myocardial infarction

103. A disease characterized by rapid abnormal production of white blood cells is:
    a. hemophilia
    b. anemia
    c. splenomegaly
    d. leukemia

104. A patient going to surgery for the removal of the spleen would sign a consent for a:
    a. spleenectomy
    b. spleenopexy
    c. splenectomy
    d. splenopexy

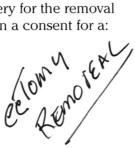

105. A patient is admitted with an inflammation of a vein as a result of a clot. The admitting diagnosis would be:
    a. thrombosis
    b. arteriothrombosis
    c. thrombophlebitis
    d. embolism

106. A cardiologist would treat which of the following conditions?
    a. hypertension
    b. uremia
    c. stomatitis
    d. hepatoma

107. A doctor's order for an x-ray of blood vessels with dye used as contrast medium is an order for a/an:
    a. angiogram
    b. aortogram
    c. arteriogram
    d. venogram

108. The process of recording electrical impulses of the heart is:
    a. electrocardiograph
    b. electrocardiography
    c. electrocardiogram
    d. electromyogram

109. A disease that attacks the immune system of patients, making them very susceptible to infection, is:
    a. CAD
    b. anemia
    c. CHF
    d. AIDS

110. A patient's H&P indicates that he has high blood pressure; the medical term for this condition is:
    a. arrhythmia
    b. hypotension
    c. hypertension
    d. tachycardia

☑ ANSWERS AND RATIONALE

98. **(d)** The blood travels from the pulmonary vein into the left atrium. p. 507

99. **(a)** Storing blood for emergency use is the function of the spleen. Its second function is to destroy old red blood cells, bacteria, and germs. p. 507

100. **(c)** Atherosclerosis is the buildup of plaque on the arterial wall. p. 507

101. **(b)** Hemorrhoids is the name given to enlarged veins in the rectal area; therefore, hemorrhoidectomy is the term used to describe surgical removal of hemorrhoids. p. 508

102. **(d)** A myocardial infarction is referred to as a heart attack. p. 507

103. **(d)** Leukemia is a disease characterized by rapid abnormal production of white blood cells. p. 513

104. **(c)** Splenectomy means surgical excision of the spleen. The word root for spleen has only one *e*, as in *splen/o*. p. 513

105. **(c)** Thrombophlebitis is the inflammation of a vein as the result of a clot. p. 513

106. **(a)** Hypertension, or high blood pressure, would be treated by a cardiologist. p. 512

107. **(a)** An angiogram is an x-ray of the blood vessel. *Angi/o* is the combining form for blood vessel. p. 513

108. **(b)** Electrocardiography is the process of recording electrical impulses of the heart. The suffix *-graphy* means process of recording, *-gram* refers to the record, and *-graph* refers to the instrument used to record. p. 513

109. **(d)** AIDS (acquired immunodeficiency syndrome) is caused by the human immunodeficiency virus (HIV), which infects certain white blood cells of the body's immune system and gradually destroys the body's ability to fight infection. p. 508

    CAD—coronary artery disease

    CHF—congestive heart failure

110. **(c)** Hypertension is the term for high blood pressure. p. 512

NOTES

UNIT 7: The Digestive System

111. Utilization of digested food by body cells is called:
  a. metabolism
  b. digestion
  c. absorption
  d. mastication

112. Mastication occurs in the:
  a. stomach
  b. mouth
  c. rectum
  d. small intestine

113. The digestive process begins with the:
  a. food entering the stomach
  b. food entering the small intestine
  c. flow of saliva into the mouth
  d. food entering the large intestine

114. Food leaving the esophagus enters the:
  a. duodenum
  b. ascending colon
  c. stomach
  d. pyloric sphincter

115. Peristalsis is:
  a. churning of food in the stomach
  b. involuntary wavelike movements
  c. process of absorption
  d. uncontrolled coughing

116. Food leaves the stomach after how many minutes?
  a. 15
  b. 30
  c. 45
  d. 60

117. Which of the following substances chemically aid digestion in the stomach?
  a. intestinal enzymes
  b. pancreatic enzymes
  c. bile
  d. hydrochloric acid

118. Which of the following is a portion of the large intestine?
  a. colon
  b. jejunum
  c. duodenum
  d. ilium

119. The small intestine is how many feet in length?
  a. 5
  b. 10
  c. 15
  d. 20

120. Digestion is completed in the:
  a. small intestine
  b. large intestine
  c. rectum
  d. stomach

121. The appendix is attached to the:
  a. ascending colon
  b. cecum
  c. sigmoid
  d. rectum

122. The function of the large intestine is:
  a. elimination
  b. mastication
  c. ingestion
  d. chemical digestion

123. Which of the following accessory organs secretes bile?
  a. liver
  b. gallbladder
  c. pancreas
  d. islets of Langerhans

124. Insulin is necessary for the metabolism of:
  a. fats
  b. carbohydrates
  c. protein
  d. fiber

125. Pancreatic enzymes and bile are released into the:
  a. jejunum
  b. ileum
  c. ilium
  d. duodenum

126. Which of the following procedures would be used to diagnose a peptic ulcer?
  a. abdominocentesis
  b. proctoscopy
  c. cholecystogram
  d. esophagogastroduodenoscopy

☑ *Answers And Rationale*

111. **(a)** Metabolism is the utilization of digested foods by the body cells. pp. 519, 521

112. **(b)** Mastication, the act of chewing food, takes place in the mouth. p. 519

113. **(c)** The digestive process begins with the flow of saliva into the mouth from the three salivary glands: parotid, submandibular, and sublingual. p. 519

114. **(c)** Food leaving the esophagus enters the stomach. The function of the esophagus is simply the passage of food. p. 519

115. **(b)** Peristalsis is the involuntary wavelike movement that propels food along the alimentary canal. p. 520

116. **(b)** Food leaves the stomach after 30 minutes. Food continues to leave the stomach at 30-minute intervals until the stomach is empty. p. 520

117. **(d)** Hydrochloric acid and gastric enzymes produced by the gastric glands located in the mucous membrane lining of the stomach chemically aid in the digestion of food. p. 520

118. **(a)** The colon is a portion of the large intestine. The jejunum and duodenum are parts of the small intestine. The ilium is a part of the pelvic bone. p. 522

119. **(d)** The small intestine is 20 feet in length and is so named because it is smaller in diameter than the large intestine. The large intestine is 5 feet in length. p. 521

120. **(a)** Digestion is completed in the small intestine, where absorption, the transfer of digested food from the small intestine to the bloodstream, takes place. p. 521

121. **(b)** The appendix, which has no function, is attached to the cecum. p. 522

122. **(a)** The function of the large intestine is elimination and also the absorption of water. p. 522

123. **(a)** The liver secretes bile, which is stored in the gallbladder. p. 522

124. **(b)** Insulin, produced by the islets of Langerhans, is necessary for the metabolism of carbohydrates. p. 522

125. **(d)** Bile, which aids in the digestion of fat, and pancreatic enzymes are released into the duodenum. p. 522

126. **(c)** An esophagogastroduodenoscopy, a visual examination of the esophagus, stomach, and duodenum, may be used for diagnosing a peptic ulcer. p. 530

NOTES

127. A patient admitted with gallstones lodged in the common bile duct would have a diagnosis of:
a. cholelithiasis
b. cholecystectomy
c. choledocholithiasis
d. Crohn's disease

128. Diverticular disease occurs:
a. on the intestinal wall
b. in the stomach lining
c. along the esophagus
d. in the mouth

129. A temporary colostomy may be performed as treatment for which of the following conditions?
a. duodenal ulcer
b. peptic ulcer
c. diverticular disease
d. cholelithiasis

130. The medical term for lesions or sores of the mucous membrane of the esophagus, stomach, or duodenum is:
a. peptic ulcer
b. diverticulitis
c. gastritis
d. ulcerative colitis

131. A patient going to surgery to have an artificial opening created in the third portion of the small intestine would sign a consent for a/an:
a. colostomy
b. ileostomy
c. gastrostomy
d. cheiloplasty

132. A patient admitted to the hospital with the diagnosis of gallstones has:
a. infectious hepatitis
b. stomatitis
c. pancreatitis
d. cholelithiasis

133. A doctor ordering an x-ray of the bile ducts would write the order for a/an:
a. cholecystogram
b. cholangiogram
c. upper GI series
d. abdominocentesis

134. The doctor wanting an x-ray of the patient's colon would order a:
a. proctoscopy
b. sigmoidoscopy
c. GI series
d. barium enema

135. A patient who is to have a visual examination of the rectum would sign a consent for a/an:
a. esophagoscopy
b. proctoscopy
c. sigmoidoscopy
d. gastroscopy

136. A patient with a tumor of the liver has:
a. glossoplegia
b. hepatoma
c. hepatomegaly
d. pancreatic

137. Which of the following procedures may be performed for treatment of ulcers?
a. abdominal herniorrhaphy
b. esophagoenterostomy
c. gastrectomy, pyloroplasty, vagotomy
d. herniorrhaphy

138. Which of the following terms means pertaining to under the tongue?
a. stomatogastric
b. sublingual
c. glossoplegia
d. proctorrhea

139. A doctor would order which procedure to aid in the diagnosis of pyloric stenosis?
a. IVP
b. GB series
c. UGI
d. BE

UNIT 8: The Respiratory System

140. External respiration is the exchange of gases between:
a. body cells and blood in the capillaries
b. the lungs and the blood
c. the nose and the external environment
d. the pulmonary artery and the pulmonary vein

☑ ANSWERS AND RATIONALE

127. **(c)** Choledocholithiasis is the condition of gallstones lodged in the common bile duct. p. 523

128. **(a)** Diverticular disease is caused by the forming of small pouches on the intestinal wall. p. 523

129. **(c)** In severe cases, a temporary colostomy may be performed as a treatment for diverticular disease. p. 523

130. **(a)** Peptic ulcer is a lesion of the mucous membrane of the esophagus, stomach (gastric ulcer), or duodenum (duodenal ulcer). p. 522

131. **(b)** Ileostomy is an artificial opening into the ileum, the third portion of the small intestine. p. 529

132. **(d)** Cholelithiasis is the condition of gallstones. p. 529

133. **(b)** A cholangiogram is an x-ray of the bile ducts. p. 530

134. **(d)** A barium enema is a procedure to x-ray the colon. p. 530

135. **(b)** Proctoscopy is the visual examination of the rectum. p. 530

136. **(b)** Hepatoma means tumor of the liver. p. 529

137. **(c)** Gastrectomy (excision of the stomach), pyloroplasty (plastic repair of the pyloric sphincter), and vagotomy (incision into the vagus nerve) are performed as a treatment for ulcers. p. 529

138. **(b)** Sublingual means pertaining to *(-al)* under *(sub-)* the tongue *(lingu/o)*. p. 529

139. **(c)** A UGI (upper gastrointestinal) examination using barium as a contrast medium would be ordered to confirm the diagnosis. p. 530

140. **(b)** External respiration is the exchange of gases between the lungs and the blood. p. 536

TEST-TAKING TIP

Do not spend more than a minute or two on a question. If you are having difficulty selecting an answer, note that you did not answer the question, move on to the next, and then return to the unanswered questions when you have completed the exam. Subsequent questions may give you a clue to the correct answer.

141. During internal respiration:
     a. body cells take on oxygen
     b. body cells take on carbon dioxide
     c. lungs take on oxygen
     d. lungs give off oxygen

142. Both food and air pass through the:
     a. larynx
     b. pharynx
     c. trachea
     d. bronchi

143. The anatomic term for the windpipe is:
     a. larynx
     b. pharynx
     c. bronchi
     d. trachea

144. The tubular structure located below the pharynx and connecting with the trachea is the:
     a. bronchi
     b. pharynx
     c. larynx
     d. bronchiole

145. Which of the following structures prevents choking?
     a. epiglottis
     b. vocal cords
     c. alveoli
     d. trachea

146. A double sac that surrounds each lung is called:
     a. alveoli
     b. pleura
     c. bronchiole
     d. pneumothorax

147. The exchange of gases that takes place in the lungs occurs between the capillaries and the:
     a. epiglottis
     b. bronchioles
     c. alveoli
     d. pleura

148. Air passes from the trachea into the:
     a. bronchioles
     b. bronchi
     c. larynx
     d. alveoli

149. A patient is admitted after an MVA with a collapsed lung. The admitting diagnosis is:
     a. pulmonary embolism
     b. hemothorax
     c. pneumothorax
     d. pleuritis

150. A pulmonary embolism is usually caused by:
     a. a virus
     b. a thrombus
     c. air
     d. a bacterium

151. Patients experiencing a temporary stoppage of breathing are said to have:
     a. apnea
     b. asthma
     c. dyspnea
     d. hyperpnea

152. A patient who has an infection of the lung has:
     a. pneumothorax
     b. pleuritis
     c. pneumonia
     d. bronchitis

153. A patient who has a nosebleed has:
     a. rhinoplasty
     b. rhinopharyngitis
     c. rhinorrhagia
     d. rhinorrhea

154. The doctor has scheduled a procedure to perform a surgical puncture and drainage of fluid from the chest cavity. The HUC would prepare a consent for a/an:
     a. abdominocentesis
     b. thoracentesis
     c. thoracotomy
     d. tracheostomy

155. An artificial opening into the windpipe is a:
     a. tracheostomy
     b. tracheotomy
     c. thoracotomy
     d. thoracentesis

156. What disease is characterized by destructive changes in the walls of the alveoli?
     a. pneumonia
     b. emphysema
     c. pleuritis
     d. asthma

☑ **ANSWERS AND RATIONALE**

141. **(a)** During internal respiration, body cells take on oxygen from the blood and at the same time give off carbon dioxide. p. 536
142. **(b)** Both food and air pass through the throat, or pharynx. p. 536
143. **(d)** The trachea, which extends from the larynx to the bronchi, is the anatomic term for the windpipe. p. 537
144. **(c)** The larynx, also known as the voice box, connects the pharynx to the trachea and contains the vocal cords, which produce sound. p. 537
145. **(a)** The epiglottis automatically covers the larynx during swallowing to prevent food from entering the larynx. p. 537
146. **(b)** The pleura is the double sac that surrounds the lung. p. 537
147. **(c)** The exchange of gases takes place between the capillaries and the one-celled wall of the alveoli. p. 536
148. **(b)** Air passes from the trachea into the bronchi. p. 537
149. **(c)** A pneumothorax is a collapsed lung resulting from the collection of air or gas in the pleural cavity. pp. 537, 538
150. **(b)** Pulmonary embolism is usually caused by a thrombus that has been dislodged from a leg vein and now blocks the pulmonary artery. p. 538
151. **(a)** Apnea is the temporary stoppage of breathing. p. 541
152. **(c)** Pneumonia is an inflammation or infection of the lung. p. 541
153. **(c)** Rhinorrhagia is another term for nosebleed (also called epistaxis). p. 542
154. **(b)** Thoracentesis is the surgical puncture and drainage of fluid from the chest cavity. p. 541
155. **(a)** A tracheostomy is the creation of an artificial opening into the windpipe. p. 541
156. **(b)** Emphysema, a degenerative disease, is characterized by destructive changes in the walls of the alveoli. p. 541

NOTES

157. Which of the following terms is spelled correctly?
    a. tonsillitis
    b. rinoplasty
    c. tonsilectomy
    d. trachesophageal

158. An x-ray image of the bronchi and the lung would require the HUC to order a:
    a. bronchitis
    b. bronchogram
    c. bronchoscope
    d. bronchoscopy

159. Excision of the voice box would require the HUC to prepare a consent for a:
    a. lobectomy
    b. laryngectomy
    c. lobotomy
    d. laryngopexy

160. Which of the following terms is spelled correctly?
    a. adenoiditis
    b. endotrakeal
    c. pulmonery
    d. bronchotrakeal

161. Paralysis of the throat is:
    a. laryngoplegia
    b. pharyngoplegia
    c. laryngopexy
    d. pharyngopexy

162. A patient admitted with a diagnosis of COPD would be admitted to which of the following units?
    a. CICU
    b. pulmonary
    c. orthopedics
    d. neurology

UNIT 9: The Urinary System and the Male Reproductive System

163. The function of the urinary system is to:
    a. produce waste material in the blood
    b. remove waste material from the blood and excrete it from the body
    c. remove waste material from the body cells
    d. transport nutrients to the cells

164. The basic unit of the kidney that removes waste material from the blood is called the:
    a. neuron
    b. nephron
    c. renal pelvis
    d. ureter

165. The tube that extends from the kidney to the bladder is called the:
    a. urethra
    b. ulna
    c. ureter
    d. urinary tube

166. The urinary bladder:
    a. produces urine
    b. adds fluid to urea
    c. provides a passageway for urine
    d. provides a container for urine

167. What percent of urine is waste material?
    a. 5%
    b. 10%
    c. 15%
    d. 20%

168. The hormone secreted by the male reproductive system is:
    a. progesterone
    b. estrogen
    c. parathormone
    d. testosterone

169. Sperm is produced in the:
    a. vas deferens
    b. urethra
    c. seminiferous tubules
    d. prostate gland

170. The epididymis is located in the:
    a. abdomen
    b. scrotum
    c. testes
    d. prostate gland

171. The prostate gland:
    a. has no function
    b. assists in the passage of urine
    c. aids in the motility of sperm
    d. aids in the production of sperm

☑ *ANSWERS AND RATIONALE*

157. **(a)** Tonsil has one "l," but the word root for tonsil is *tonsill(o)*; therefore, tonsillitis has two "l's." p. 541

158. **(b)** A bronchogram is an x-ray image of the bronchi and lung. p. 542

159. **(b)** A laryngectomy is the excision of the voice box. p. 541

160. **(a)** The correct spelling is adenoiditis. p. 541

161. **(b)** Pharyngoplegia is paralysis of the throat. p. 541

162. **(b)** A patient having a diagnosis of COPD (chronic obstructive pulmonary disease) would be admitted to the pulmonary unit. p. 541

163. **(b)** The function of the urinary system, also called the excretory system, is to remove waste from the blood and excrete it from the body. p. 546

164. **(b)** Over 1 million nephrons located in each kidney are made up of a system of arteries, capillaries, and tubules. Their function is to remove waste material from the blood. p. 546

165. **(c)** The ureter, approximately 10 to 12 inches in length, extends from each kidney to the urinary bladder. It provides a passageway for urine. pp. 546, 547

166. **(d)** The urinary bladder is the container for urine. p. 547

167. **(a)** Approximately 5% of urine is waste material; the remainder is water. The daily amount produced by the kidney is 1500 mL. p. 547

168. **(d)** Testosterone is secreted by the testicles and is responsible for the development of the male secondary sex characteristics. p. 548

169. **(c)** Sperm is produced in the seminiferous tubules. p. 548

170. **(b)** The epididymis is a tiny 20-inch tube located in the scrotum atop the testicle. p. 548

171. **(c)** The prostate gland secretes a fluid that aids in the motility of sperm. p. 548

NOTES

172. The term that means pertaining to urine is:
   a. urination
   b. urinary
   c. urology
   d. void

173. A patient admitted to the hospital with the diagnosis of renal calculi has:
   a. pyelonephritis
   b. uremia
   c. nephritis
   d. nephrolithiasis

174. A patient is scheduled for an excision of one or both testes will undergo a/an:
   a. orchiectomy
   b. prostatectomy
   c. circumcision
   d. vasectomy

175. Urethrorrhaphy means:
   a. suture of a urethral tear
   b. plastic repair of the urethra
   c. removal of a stone
   d. hemorrhage from the urethra

176. Which of the following terms is spelled correctly?
   a. urologest
   b. uralogy
   c. ureteralgea
   d. scrotum

177. Incision into the kidney to remove a stone is:
   a. nephrectomy
   b. nephropexy
   c. nephrolithotomy
   d. nephrolithiasis

178. A patient with urine in the blood has:
   a. hematuria
   b. uremia
   c. hydrocele
   d. cystocele

179. Scheduling a patient for removal of a portion of the prostate would require the HUC to prepare a consent for a/an:
   a. prostatomy
   b. transurethral resection
   c. orchiectomy
   d. prostatolith

180. A laboratory test used to determine kidney function is:
   a. hemoglobin
   b. urinalysis
   c. blood urea nitrogen
   d. hematocrit

181. The medical term for a visual examination of the bladder is:
   a. cystogram
   b. cystoscopy
   c. cystography
   d. cystoscope

182. A patient with an inflammation of the bladder has:
   a. nephritis
   b. cystocele
   c. cystitis
   d. nephrolithiasis

UNIT 10: The Female Reproductive System

183. Which of the following is a function of the female reproductive system?
   a. produce sperm
   b. produce insulin
   c. provide for conception
   d. excrete waste

184. The main body of the uterus is called the:
   a. cervix
   b. fundus
   c. vagina
   d. endometrium

185. The female reproductive cell, or ovum, is produced by the:
   a. ovaries
   b. uterus
   c. fallopian tube
   d. vagina

186. Fertilization usually takes place in the:
   a. fallopian tube
   b. uterus
   c. vagina
   d. ovaries

☑ *ANSWERS AND RATIONALE*

172. **(b)** Urinary means pertaining to urine. p. 551

173. **(d)** Renal calculi and nephrolithiasis are both medical terms for kidney stones. p. 552

174. **(a)** Orchiectomy means excision of one or both testes. p. 551

175. **(a)** Urethrorrhaphy means suture of a urethral tear. p. 551

176. **(d)** The correct spelling is scrotum. p. 547

177. **(c)** Nephrolithotomy is the incision into the kidney to remove a stone. p. 551

178. **(b)** Uremia is urine in the blood. p. 552

179. **(b)** Transurethral resection is surgery performed to remove a portion of the prostate gland through the urethra. p. 551

180. **(c)** Blood urea nitrogen (BUN) is a laboratory test used to determine kidney function. p. 552

181. **(b)** Cystoscopy is the visual examination of the bladder. p. 552

182. **(c)** Cystitis is inflammation of the bladder. p. 552

183. **(d)** Providing for conception is a function of the female reproductive system. p. 556

184. **(b)** The main body of the uterus is called the fundus. p. 556

185. **(a)** The ovum is produced by the ovaries. p. 556

186. **(a)** Fertilization usually takes place in the fallopian tube. p. 557

NOTES

187. Estrogen and progesterone are produced by the:
a. ovaries
b. fallopian tubes
c. uterus
d. vagina

188. The hormone progesterone helps in the:
a. menstrual cycle
b. development of female reproductive organs
c. development of breasts
d. preparation of the uterus for conception and pregnancy

189. The muscular tube, 3 inches in length, that connects the uterus to the outside of the body is the:
a. urethra
b. rectum
c. vagina
d. uterine tube

190. The perineum is the:
a. base of the uterus
b. lateral portion of the buttocks
c. area between the vaginal opening and the anus
d. area of the pelvic floor anterior to the meatus

191. The medical term that means "without menstrual discharge" is:
a. metrorrhagia
b. dysmenorrhea
c. amenorrhea
d. metrorrhea

192. Which of the following terms is spelled correctly?
a. gynacologist
b. gynacology
c. ureterovaginal
d. utarine

193. A patient scheduled for a hysterosalpingo-oophorectomy will be having a surgical removal of the:
a. ovaries, uterus, and fallopian tubes
b. ovaries, uterus, and cervix
c. fallopian tubes, uterus, and vagina
d. ureter, ovaries, and fallopian tubes

194. The surgical procedure to scrape the inner walls of the uterus is a:
a. colporrhaphy
b. dilation and curettage
c. perineorrhaphy
d. hysterectomy

195. Cervicectomy is the medical term for:
a. inflammation of the cervix
b. excision of the cervix
c. incision of the cervix
d. x-ray image of the cervix

196. Which of the following is spelled correctly?
a. menopause
b. menstural
c. vaginel
d. mensturation

197. A patient scheduled for the removal of an ovary would sign a consent for a/an:
a. oophorectomy
b. salpingectomy
c. salpingo-oophorectomy
d. hysterectomy

198. The medical term that means visual examination of the vagina is:
a. vaginal speculum
b. colposcopy
c. colposcope
d. cervical Pap smear

199. A patient admitted with a diagnosis of a salpingocele has a/an:
a. herniation of the fallopian tube
b. herniation of the ovary
c. inflammation of the fallopian tube
d. inflammation of the ovary

200. Which of the following terms means "pertaining to birth"?
a. natal
b. neonatal
c. postnatal
d. prenatal

201. Which of the following terms is spelled correctly?
a. obstetrician
b. obstretics
c. aborshun
d. amniotec fluid

☑ ANSWERS AND RATIONALE

187. **(a)** Estrogen and progesterone are produced by the ovaries. p. 557

188. **(d)** Progesterone helps in preparing the uterus for conception and pregnancy. p. 557

189. **(c)** The vagina connects the uterus to the outside of the body. p. 557

190. **(c)** The pelvic floor of both the male and the female is called the perineum; the term is also used to describe the area between the vaginal opening and the anus of the female. p. 557

191. **(c)** Amenorrhea means without menstrual discharge. p. 561

192. **(c)** Ureterovaginal is the correct spelling. p. 561

193. **(a)** Hysterosalpingo-oophorectomy is the surgical removal of the ovaries, uterus, and fallopian tubes. p. 562

194. **(b)** Dilation and curettage (D & C) is the surgical procedure to scrape the inner walls of the uterus. p. 561

195. **(b)** Cervicectomy means excision of the cervix. p. 561

196. **(a)** Menopause is the correct spelling. p. 561

197. **(a)** Oophorectomy is the surgical removal of the ovary. p. 561

198. **(b)** Colposcopy is the visual examination of the vagina and cervix. p. 562

199. **(a)** Salpingocele is the herniation of the fallopian tube. p. 562

200. **(a)** Natal means pertaining to birth. p. 565

201. **(a)** Obstetrician is the correct spelling. p. 565

NOTES

202. The medical term that means "present at birth" is:
   a. fetus
   b. congenital
   c. placenta
   d. genetic

203. A GYN patient admitted because of an ectopic pregnancy has a:
   a. fertilized ovum implanted outside of the uterus
   b. fertilized ovum implanted inside the uterus
   c. fertilized ovum implanted in the ovary
   d. fertilized ovum implanted in the vagina

UNIT 11: The Endocrine System

204. Which of the following is a function of the endocrine system?
   a. connection and control
   b. control and communication
   c. communication and circulation
   d. none of the above

205. Endocrine secretions go directly into the:
   a. ducts
   b. glands
   c. bloodstream
   d. brain

206. Which of the following is often referred to as the master gland?
   a. pituitary
   b. adrenal
   c. thyroid
   d. sebaceous

207. Which of the following hormones is produced by the posterior lobe of the pituitary gland?
   a. ADH
   b. TSH
   c. GH
   d. ACTH

208. Which of the following stimulates contraction of the uterus during childbirth?
   a. thyroxin
   b. oxytocin
   c. parathormone
   d. prolactin

209. Iodine is necessary in the body for the production of:
   a. thyroxin
   b. oxytocin
   c. antidiuretic hormone
   d. epinephrine

210. The hormone necessary for the metabolism of carbohydrates is:
   a. erythropoietin
   b. thyroxin
   c. insulin
   d. parathormone

211. Epinephrine is produced by which of the following glands?
   a. adrenal cortex
   b. adrenal medulla
   c. thyroid
   d. parathyroid

212. The amount of calcium in the blood is regulated by which of the following glands?
   a. parathyroid
   b. thyroid
   c. adrenal
   d. pituitary

213. Which of the following hormones maintains metabolism of body cells?
   a. thyroxin
   b. oxytocin
   c. epinephrine
   d. norepinephrine

214. Excessive insulin in the blood may cause:
   a. diabetic coma
   b. convulsions
   c. insulin shock
   d. extreme thirst

215. Fasting blood sugar is used to diagnose:
   a. diabetes mellitus
   b. diabetes insipidus
   c. Graves' disease
   d. Addison's disease

216. Which of the following medical terms means "abnormal condition of a gland"?
   a. adenitis
   b. adenoid
   c. adenoma
   d. adenosis

✔ ANSWERS AND RATIONALE

202. **(b)** Congenital means present at birth. p. 565

203. **(a)** An ectopic pregnancy is a fertilized ovum implanted outside of the uterus. p. 565

204. **(b)** The function of the endocrine system is similar to that of the nervous system: to communicate and to control. p. 567

205. **(c)** Endocrine glands are ductless glands and do not have tubes to carry secretions to other parts of the body. The secretions go directly into the bloodstream. p. 567

206. **(a)** The pituitary gland is referred to as the master gland because it produces hormones that stimulate function of the other endocrine glands. p. 568

207. **(a)** ADH is produced by the posterior lobe of the pituitary gland. p. 568

208. **(b)** Oxytocin, produced by the anterior lobe of the pituitary gland, stimulates contraction of the uterus during childbirth. p. 568

209. **(a)** Iodine is necessary in the body for the production of thyroxin. p. 568

210. **(c)** Insulin is necessary for the metabolism of carbohydrates in the body. p. 568

211. **(b)** Epinephrine is produced by the adrenal medulla. p. 568

212. **(a)** Parathormone, produced by the parathyroid glands, regulates the amount of calcium in the blood. p. 568

213. **(a)** Thyroxin, produced by the thyroid gland, maintains metabolism of body cells. p. 568

214. **(c)** Excessive insulin in the blood may cause insulin shock, whereas too much sugar in the blood may cause diabetic coma. p. 568

215. **(a)** The fasting blood sugar is a laboratory test that determines the amount of sugar in the blood after fasting. It is used to diagnose diabetes mellitus. pp. 569, 571

216. **(d)** Adenosis means abnormal condition of a gland. p. 571

NOTES

217. Which of the following diseases is caused by lack of production of hormones by the adrenal gland?
   a. Cushing's disease
   b. diabetes mellitus
   c. diabetes insipidus
   d. Addison's disease

218. Another name for hyperthyroidism is:
   a. hypothyroidism
   b. Graves' disease
   c. Cushing's disease
   d. Addison's disease

219. A disease caused by inadequate antidiuretic hormone production is:
   a. diabetes insipidus
   b. diabetes mellitus
   c. Cushing's disease
   d. Graves' disease

Inadequ

☑ ANSWERS AND RATIONALE

217. **(d)** Addison's disease is caused by lack of production of hormones by the adrenal glands. p. 571

218. **(b)** Graves' disease is another name for hyperthyroidism. pp. 569, 571

219. **(a)** Diabetes insipidus is caused by inadequate antidiuretic hormone production. p. 571

TEST-TAKING TIP

An option may be chosen on an impulse and then on review the option is changed. Avoid this. Studies have shown that the first answer that comes to mind is usually right.

Health Unit Coordinator Employment-Related Situations and Additional Questions

CHAPTER 24

Health Unit Coordinator Employment-Related Situations

The questions in this chapter cover work-related situations dealing with information that may not be specifically covered in the textbook *Health Unit Coordinating*. They are intended to measure your problem-solving and decision-making abilities. *Health Unit Coordinating* does provide a foundation of knowledge including communication and problem-solving techniques that will be helpful in answering the questions included in this chapter.

1. Dr. M. Hart is a cardiologist and attending doctor for patient Les Breath. Dr. P. Neumon, a consulting pulmonary specialist, wrote an order to transfer patient Les Breath out of CCU. To process this transfer you would (first):
   a. report the new room number to Dr. Hart's office
   b. call admitting for a bed assignment
   c. prepare the patient's chart for transfer
   d. confirm the order with Dr. Hart

2. The hospitalist wrote an order to obtain records from another hospital from a patient's previous admission, you would:
   a. contact the patient's doctor to obtain the patient's signature on an information release form and to request the records
   b. obtain the patient's signature on an information release form, fax the form to the health records department at the other hospital after calling to request records
   c. obtain the patient's signature on an information release form and notify the admissions clerk
   d. just call health care records at the other hospital and ask them to fax the patient's records

3. An order for quantitative fecal fat would require you to:
   a. send a requisition to chemistry
   b. request a stool collection container for quantitative fecal fat from the laboratory department
   c. obtain a stool specimen container for quantitative fecal fat from SPD
   d. tell the nurse to obtain a stool specimen container for quantitative fecal fat from the floor supply closet

☑ *ANSWERS AND RATIONALE*

1. **(d)** The order should be confirmed with Dr. M. Hart because Dr. P. Neumon is the consulting doctor. The patient's attending doctor is Dr. M. Hart.

2. **(b)** The patient's signature on an information release form is needed to obtain records from another hospital. Obtain the patient's signature on an information release form and fax the form to the health records department at the other hospital after calling to request records.

3. **(b)** An order for a 24- to 72-hour specimen would require a collection container from the laboratory. It is vital that, when requesting a collection container from the laboratory, you specify the test to be done so the laboratory personnel may include any additives necessary.

NOTES

4. The surgeon has written an NPO 2400 hrs order for a patient who is having an open reduction of the right femur at 1330 tomorrow. An hour later the anesthesiologist came by to write pre-op orders and ordered a clear liquid breakfast at 0600, then NPO. You would:
   a. order the NPO 2400 hrs and ignore the second order
   b. check with the surgery department
   c. order the clear liquid breakfast, then NPO as written in second order
   d. call the surgeon to clarify the order

5. You have repeatedly observed a young resident taking medical supplies from the nursing unit supply closet. He has asked you to keep quiet when he noticed that you observed this. You would:
   a. report the incidents to the nurse manager
   b. do nothing, it's not your concern
   c. advise the resident that next time you will report him
   d. call security

6. It is 2000 and the diagnostic imaging department is closed. A doctor has written an order for a stat KUB for a patient with severe abdominal pain. You would:
   a. tell the charge nurse of the situation
   b. leave the order for the next day
   c. page the diagnostic imaging technician on call
   d. do all other orders and wait until there are more diagnostic imaging orders before calling someone in for one order

7. A CBC was ordered on the wrong patient. The results came back with an elevated WBC. You would:
   a. place the results in the chart of the patient with the elevated WBC and order the CBC on the correct patient
   b. order the CBC on the correct patient and discard the CBC results that were done in error
   c. call results to the doctor of the patient with the elevated WBC with the explanation that the CBC was done by mistake, then order the CBC on the correct patient
   d. call the doctor who ordered the test and explain the situation

8. A patient is hemorrhaging, and the nurse asks you to call the blood bank to check on the unit of blood that was ordered for the patient. A doctor arrives at the same time and asks you to help him locate a patient's chart, and a visitor is asking for the location of a patient who was transferred to another unit. You would:
   a. tell the doctor and the visitor that you don't have time help them and place the call to the blood bank
   b. obtain lab results for the doctor, find the patient location for the visitor, then call the blood bank
   c. ask the nurse what to do
   d. advise the doctor and the visitor that you have a call to make and then you will be glad to assist them

9. There is a fire in the visitor's lounge that has been reported. Your reaction would be to:
   a. evacuate patients from the nursing unit
   b. close all patient doors
   c. collect and remove all charts from the nursing unit
   d. do nothing; your job is nonclinical

10. A medical student in a teaching hospital wrote orders on a newly admitted patient. The hospital policy states that medical students may not write orders. You would:
    a. page the appropriate resident to cosign the orders
    b. call the patient's attending doctor to verify the orders
    c. transcribe the orders
    d. ask the patient's nurse to cosign the orders

11. A doctor wrote orders on a patient and forgot to sign them. It is a hospital policy that orders must be signed prior to being acted upon. You would:
    a. transcribe the orders and ask the doctor to sign them the next time she makes rounds
    b. ask the patient's nurse to cosign them
    c. wait to transcribe the orders until they are signed
    d. advise the patient's nurse that you are calling the doctor so he or she can verify the orders and sign them

☑ *ANSWERS AND RATIONALE*

4. **(c)** Order the clear liquid breakfast, then NPO as written because the anesthesiologist's order would take priority over the first order.

5. **(a)** Report the incidents to the nurse manager. Missing supplies are charged to the nursing unit.

6. **(c)** Page the diagnostic imaging technician on call. There is always a technician on call for emergency situations.

7. **(c)** Call the results to the patient's doctor and then order the CBC on the correct patient. An incident report would also need to be completed.

8. **(d)** Advise the doctor and the visitor that you have a phone call to make and then you will be glad to assist them.

9. **(b)** Closing all patient doors is the fire code policy. (Be aware of fire and disaster policies.)

10. **(a)** Page the appropriate resident to cosign the orders. (Be aware of residents' patient assignments and schedules.)

11. **(d)** Advise the patient's nurse that you are placing a call to the doctor. The nurse can verify the orders and sign them, and the doctor can add her signature the next day.

NOTES

12. A doctor calls out an order to you (in a nonemergency situation) as he or she is leaving the nursing station. You would:
    a. advise the doctor that you cannot take verbal orders in nonemergency situations and ask him or her to write the order
    b. write the order as given and assume that the doctor will add his signature the next time he makes rounds
    c. write the order down and ask the patient's nurse to write the order in the chart
    d. ignore the order as he should know better than to give you verbal orders

13. A hard copy of an order refers to:
    a. the original written doctor's order
    b. the pharmacy copy of the orders
    c. a duplicate copy of the order from the computer printer
    d. phone orders written by the nurse

14. A nurse calls out to you to call a code arrest on a patient who has a living will and a written DNR order. You would:
    a. call the code anyway
    b. remind the nurse of the living will and DNR order
    c. call the patient's doctor
    d. refuse to call the code

15. A child is admitted to the ER accompanied by a babysitter. The parents (legal guardians) cannot be reached and the child needs immediate surgery to save her life. What would be done?
    a. the surgery would be delayed until the parents can be reached
    b. the child would have surgery immediately without consent
    c. two doctors would sign the consent for surgery
    d. the babysitter, without legal permission, would be asked to sign the consent

16. A patient tells you that the nurse assigned to him or her has been very rude. You would:
    a. report the complaint to the patient's nurse
    b. report the complaint to the nurse manager
    c. place a call to the patient's doctor
    d. do nothing; patients aren't your responsibility

17. A patient who is a known alcoholic and a frequent patient on your nursing unit is readmitted. His family tells you that he is complaining of a severe headache and they observe a difference in his speech. When you report this to his nurse, she states, "He is probably drunk." The patient's family approaches the nurse's station again and tells you that they are very concerned, so you again report this to the nurse and ask her to please check the patient and speak to the family. The nurse tells you to stick to your job and she will do patient care. You would:
    a. call the doctor
    b. report the incident to the nurse manager
    c. do nothing—"stick to your job"
    d. tell the family that you have done all you can

18. A patient is scheduled for surgery and has signed the surgery consent. Now the patient tells you that she has concerns about pictures being taken during surgery. You would:
    a. advise the patient's nurse
    b. call the hospital photographer
    c. call the doctor
    d. tell her that pictures probably won't be taken

19. A patient has signed a consent for a reconstructive surgery but tells you that she is having doubts and would like a second opinion. An appropriate response would be:
    a. tell her "all patient's have second thoughts, don't worry"
    b. call surgery and cancel the surgery
    c. call a priest to counsel her
    d. advise her nurse and doctor

20. A patient has been discharged and the doctor asks you to do her a favor and keep the chart on the nursing station until tomorrow so she can finish the summary sheet. You would:
    a. do as asked and keep the chart on the unit
    b. advise her that you can't do that and that she can finish the summary sheet in health records
    c. send the chart to health records and tell her you forgot
    d. ask the nurse if that would be okay

☑ *ANSWERS AND RATIONALE*

12. **(a)** Advise the doctor that hospital policy prohibits you from taking verbal orders in nonemergency situations. Ask him or her to write the order.

13. **(c)** A hard copy of an order refers to the duplicate copy of the order from the computer printer.

14. **(b)** Remind the nurse of the living will and DNR (do not resuscitate order).

15. **(c)** Two doctors can sign a surgery consent in a life-threatening emergency. The babysitter could not sign the consent unless provided with a document granting him or her the parents' legal permission to act as the child's legal guardian in an emergency.

16. **(a)** Report the complaint to the patient's nurse. Follow the chain of command; there may have been a misunderstanding that was interpreted as rudeness.

17. **(b)** Report the incident to the nurse manager. The nurse manager would be the next person in the chain of command, and the patient's welfare is the top priority.

18. **(a)** Advise the patient's nurse, who would take the surgery consent back to the patient so that she can cross out permission to photograph and initial it.

19. **(d)** Advise her nurse and doctor that the patient has concerns.

20. **(b)** Advise her that you can't do that and that she can finish the summary sheet in health records. The health records department has a limited time to complete discharge charts and to submit billing to insurance companies.

NOTES

21. When a patient expires, you would call:
    a. only the attending doctor
    b. the chief of staff
    c. all doctors involved with the patient's care
    d. the clergy on call

22. A patient's mother has been staying with her son around the clock and tells you that she has not eaten and has no money. What would be your most appropriate response?
    a. loan her some money
    b. do nothing
    c. call social services
    d. give her some food from the unit dietary kitchen

23. You had asked for a weekend off 2 months ago, but when the schedule comes out, you are scheduled to work. Your best solution would be to:
    a. tell the nurse manager when he or she comes by the nursing station
    b. work the weekend and forget your plans
    c. trade weekends with coworkers and don't involve staffing
    d. take a copy of the request to staffing and tell them there is an error

24. A patient was just told by his doctor that he has terminal cancer. The patient stops by the nursing station and tells you that he is scared and does not want to die. An appropriate response would be to:
    a. listen with empathy
    b. call a priest or pastor
    c. refer him to his nurse
    d. tell him to talk to his family

25. A patient tells you that her doctor told her that she has diabetes. She tells you that she is very confused about the severity of her illness and the treatment. Your best response would be to:
    a. look in the chart and answer her questions as much as possible
    b. call the diabetic nurse to talk to her
    c. tell her to wait until her doctor returns to get more information
    d. advise her that you will ask her nurse to come in to talk with her

26. You observe a visitor entering an isolation room without a gown and mask. Your best action would be to:
    a. ask the visitor if he or she can read signs
    b. do nothing; it's not your concern
    c. tell the nurse
    d. advise the visitor that a gown and mask has to be worn while visiting the patient

27. A consultation order is written for Dr. John Smith to see a patient regarding a ruptured disc. When obtaining a phone number from the doctor's roster, you find three Dr. John Smiths listed. You would:
    a. call the attending to clarify which Dr. Smith he or she meant
    b. call the Dr. Smith who is an orthopedist
    c. call the Dr. Smith who is an ophthalmologist
    d. call the Dr. Smith who is a geriatrist

28. You are transcribing a set of orders and you are unable to read one of the orders. The patient's nurse interprets it one way and another nurse interprets it another. You would:
    a. ask another health unit coordinator what he or she thinks
    b. ask a third nurse for interpretation
    c. assume the patient's nurse would be correct
    d. call the doctor for clarification

29. You observe a coworker adding a decimal point to a medication dose on the MAR to cover an error. The medication nurse has already given the incorrect dose. You would:
    a. wait to see if the error is discovered or if any harm is done
    b. call risk management
    c. report the incident to the nurse manager
    d. call the patient's doctor

30. You walk into a patient's room and observe an orderly treating an elderly patient in an extremely rough manner. You would:
    a. notify the nurse manager
    b. call security
    c. advise the orderly that if you ever witness another incident, you will report it
    d. do nothing; patient care is not a health unit coordinator's concern

☑ ANSWERS AND RATIONALE

21. **(c)** All doctors involved with the patient's care should be notified.

22. **(c)** Call social services, who could help her find a place to stay, if needed, and follow up with other needs.

23. **(d)** Take a copy of your request to staffing and tell them that an error was made. The request may have been overlooked. Taking the problem to the nurse manager could cause hard feelings. Follow the chain of command.

24. **(a)** Listening with empathy is the best choice. It may be okay to suggest the other options, but just listening and caring is important because the patient chose you to share his concerns and feelings.

25. **(d)** Advise her that you will ask her nurse to come in to talk with her. The patient's nurse would know the most about the diagnosis and proposed treatment. Also advise the patient to make a list of concerns and questions for her doctor.

26. **(d)** Advise the visitor of the isolation rules. It is part of the health unit coordinator's responsibilities to advise visitors of hospital rules.

27. **(b)** Call the Dr. John Smith who is an orthopedist, who treats diseases or fractures of the musculoskeletal system.

28. **(d)** Call the doctor for clarification. Don't assume anything. Question orders, policies, and procedures that do not seem appropriate.

29. **(c)** Report the incident to the nurse manager.

30. **(a)** Notify the nurse manager.

NOTES

31. A patient has signed his surgery consent. The morning of the scheduled surgery, the doctor changed the wording for the procedure to be done on the patient's order sheet. The patient has not yet been sedated. You would:
    a. change the wording for the procedure on the signed consent using White-Out
    b. prepare a new consent with the new wording and give it to the nurse for the patient to sign
    c. change the wording on the signed consent using a line drawn through the incorrect wording
    d. change the wording on the signed consent and ask the doctor to initial it

32. You are working on a busy pediatrics unit and have been assigned a student health unit coordinator to train during his or her clinical rotation. The student has made numerous errors while transcribing patient orders and does not seem competent. You would:
    a. wait another week to see if the situation improves
    b. refuse to allow the student to transcribe patient's orders, but allow him or her to observe until the clinical rotation has ended
    c. advise the student's instructor or the nurse manager right away
    d. just recheck all orders that the student transcribes, correct the errors, and say nothing

33. A hospital transport employee arrives on your nursing unit to deliver an ordered narcotic from the pharmacy. All of the RNs are busy and in patient rooms. You would:
    a. ask transport to leave the narcotic and you will have an RN sign the acceptance form later
    b. ask transport to wait for an RN to sign for the narcotic
    c. sign for the narcotic yourself
    d. ask one of the doctors to sign for the narcotic

34. You observe a coworker acting in a very strange manner and detect a smell of alcohol on his or her breath. You would:
    a. mind your business and do nothing
    b. advise the nurse manager
    c. call security and report the situation
    d. advise the coworker to go home

35. A patient on your unit is being kept alive by life support. A family member approaches you at the nurse's station to ask how you would feel about removing the life support. You would:
    a. advise the family member to talk to the doctor about it
    b. tell the family member that you are not allowed to talk about that
    c. tell the family member how you feel about life support
    d. call the hospital priest

36. A coworker has admitted to you that he or she has a serious drug problem but does not plan on reporting or correcting the problem. The coworker is in a position that could place patients at risk. You would:
    a. wait to see if the coworker will seek help
    b. advise security
    c. do nothing and respect the coworker's confidence
    d. advise the nurse manager

37. A patient on your unit has been transferred to an ECF. After the patient has gone, you realize that you sent the original patient records rather than the copies. You would:
    a. call the ECF and advise them of the error
    b. call the patient's family and ask them to return the originals immediately
    c. place the copies in the chart to health records and say nothing
    d. call health records to report the error immediately

38. When transcribing a doctor's order for ampicillin, you observe on the MAR that the patient is allergic to PCN. You would:
    a. transcribe the order; the doctor must know the patient's allergies
    b. call the pharmacy
    c. notify the doctor of the patient's allergy
    d. ask the patient if he or she is allergic to ampicillin

✔ **ANSWERS AND RATIONALE**

31. **(b)** A change in the procedure would require a new consent form, and the patient would have to be informed of the procedure, including its risks and characteristics (informed consent).

32. **(c)** Advise the student's instructor or the nurse manager right away.

33. **(b)** Ask transport to wait for an RN to sign for the narcotic. An RN must sign for a narcotic delivered to the nursing unit.

34. **(b)** Advise the nurse manager of the incident.

35. **(a)** Advise the family member to discuss removing the patient from life support with the doctor.

36. **(d)** Advise the nurse manager. The patients' safety must come first.

37. **(d)** Call health records and report the error immediately.

38. **(c)** Notify the doctor of the patient's allergy.

TEST TAKING TIP

Answer all questions, because the scoring is the same whether you answer incorrectly or not at all, and you might select the correct answer.

39. There are two charts in the chart rack with a red tape on each of the chart spines marked "name alert." This would indicate that:
    a. the patient's names are difficult to spell
    b. the two patients are related
    c. the two patients have the same last name
    d. the two patients share the same doctor

40. You are working in a PICU and receive a call from one of the pediatric floor units that you are receiving a patient who just coded. All the nurses on the unit are unable to leave their patients or are at lunch. You would:
    a. page the nurse manager
    b. call one of the other units to ask for help
    c. tell the floor unit to hold the patient until a nurse returns from lunch
    d. advise the floor unit to bring the patient and you will try to assist the doctors if necessary

41. A doctor has made sexually intimidating remarks to you. You have asked him or her to stop, but he or she persists in making advances. You would:
    a. avoid contact with the doctor as much as possible and say nothing
    b. report the situation to security
    c. the next time a remark is made, slap him or her
    d. report the situation to the nurse manager

42. A doctor has written an order for a surgery consent. You are not sure of the spelling of the procedure. You would:
    a. check the spelling on the surgery schedule
    b. ask one of the nurses
    c. check the spelling in the medical dictionary
    d. call the doctor to obtain correct spelling

43. An order has been written to have a blood transfusion consent signed by the parent of a child going to surgery. You advise the nurse and he or she asks you to tell the parents not to leave so the consent can be signed. You would:
    a. just tell the parents to stay on the unit without any explanation
    b. advise the parents that the nurse has a form that needs to be signed and to please remain on the unit
    c. ignore the request because the parents are always there anyway
    d. advise the parents that a blood transfusion consent needs to be signed

44. When calling a code on a pediatric unit, you should instruct the switchboard operator to:
    a. state pediatric code
    b. indicate nonadult code
    c. call for all pediatricians to come to the unit stat
    d. call a code just as any other code

45. A patient with which of the following diagnoses on a pediatric unit would need to be in isolation?
    a. RAD
    b. RSV
    c. FTT
    d. SNAT

46. Central service supply discrepancies are absorbed by the:
    a. recently discharged patients
    b. patients currently on the nursing unit
    c. central service department
    d. individual nursing units

47. An incident report is initiated if a nurse:
    a. accidentally takes the narcotics cabinet keys home with him or her
    b. goes to the hospital cafeteria with the narcotic cabinet keys
    c. leaves the nursing unit with the narcotics cabinet keys
    d. is late administering a narcotic to a patient

☑ *ANSWERS AND RATIONALE*

39. **(c)** The two patients have the same last name. This type of labeling is done to avoid errors in ordering tests and procedures and filing reports.

40. **(a)** Page the nurse manager.

41. **(d)** Report the situation to the nurse manager. No one has to tolerate sexual harassment.

42. **(c)** Check the spelling in the medical dictionary.

43. **(b)** Advise the parents that the nurse has a form that needs to be signed and to please remain on the unit. The nurse will explain the need for the blood transfusion consent to the parent.

44. **(a)** A specialized pediatric code team, including the pediatric intensivist, will respond to a pediatric code. (This may not apply if you are working in a smaller hospital that would not have pediatric specialists.)

45. **(b)** RSV (respiratory syncytial virus) is a particular risk to patients who have lung dysfunction (e.g., bronchial pulmonary dysplasia, reactive airway disease).

RAD—reactive airway disease
FTT—failure to thrive
SNAT—suspected nonaccidental trauma (abuse)

46. **(d)** Central service supply discrepancies are absorbed by the individual nursing units. The health unit coordinator may be involved in finding lost charges to reduce cost to nursing unit.

47. **(a)** An incident report is initiated if a nurse accidentally goes home with the narcotics cabinet keys. A locksmith will be called to change the narcotics cabinet lock.

NOTES

48. An order for a chest PA and LAT this AM was overlooked and discovered at 3:30 PM. You would:
    a. order the x-ray stat
    b. order the x-ray for the next day in the AM
    c. do nothing because it was not your error
    d. order the x-ray ASAP and notify patient's nurse

49. The HUC on the day shift is related to one of the doctors and constantly leaves excess work for you to do. You have found orders that were written in the AM when you arrive at 3:00 PM. You talked with him or her about this, but the situation has gotten worse. You would:
    a. talk to the nurse manager
    b. refuse to transcribe orders written before noon
    c. talk to the HUC again
    d. do nothing; the nurse manager must be aware and does not want to get involved

50. While working on a busy medical unit, a doctor asks you to find out when a CT that she has ordered will be done, a nurse asks you to order a floatation mattress for a patient who has pressure sores, a visitor is asking for visitation information, and the unit phone is ringing. Which task would you respond to first?
    a. the doctor's, because they always have priority
    b. the nurse's request for a floatation mattress, because the patient's welfare should come first
    c. the visitor's questions, because it would be good public relations put visitors' needs first
    d. the ringing telephone, because there could be an urgent situation

51. A family member of a discharged geriatric patient confides in you that there is neglect and abuse happening in the patient's home and she fears for the patient's safety. You would:
    a. do nothing because it is not your place to get involved
    b. advise the patient's nurse of what has been told to you
    c. call a social worker and report what you have been told
    d. place a stat call to the patient's doctor

52. It is the middle of winter and very cold. A pediatric patient has a discharge order written. The child's mother tells you that the electricity has been shut off because she did not have money to pay the bill. You would:
    a. tell her that she will need to find the money for her child's sake
    b. give her the money if you can afford it
    c. call the electric company, explain the situation, and ask them to turn the electricity back on
    d. advise the patient's nurse of what you were told

53. While working on a pediatric unit, you observe a mother on two separate occasions leaving a siderail halfway down on her 10-month-old child's crib as she was leaving the room. On both occasions, you reminded her of the danger that the child could easily fall over the rail onto the floor. The next day, you are told that the child fell over the side rail and that an incident report had been made out. You would:
    a. remind the mother of the previous incidents
    b. say nothing—accidents happen
    c. report the previous incidents to the patient's nurse
    d. call the patient's doctor to report the previous incidents

54. The husband of a patient arrives on the unit with his two children insisting that they be allowed to see their mother, who is close to death. Rules on that unit prohibit children from visiting. You would:
    a. sneak the children in to visit their mother
    b. explain that hospital rules prohibit the children from visiting
    c. call the nurse manager and explain the situation
    d. call security

55. You receive a call informing you of a critical blood gas report on a patient. What would you do first?
    a. notify the patient's nurse
    b. page the resident
    c. go to the patient's room and notify the family
    d. call the patient's doctor

☑ ANSWERS AND RATIONALE

48. **(d)** Order the x-ray ASAP and notify the patient's nurse. Procedures are only ordered stat if the doctor writes an order for them to be done stat.

49. **(a)** Talk to the nurse manager about the problem, because patients' orders must be transcribed within a reasonable time.

50. **(d)** The ringing telephone always takes priority. You would excuse yourself to the doctor, nurse, and visitor, and address their requests after answering the phone.

51. **(b)** The patient's nurse should be told first. He or she may ask you to place a call to the social worker, but chain of command would require that the nurse to be informed first.

52. **(d)** Advise the patient's nurse, who may ask you to place a call to the case manager or social worker.

53. **(c)** Report the previous incidents to the patient's nurse, who may advise you to call risk management to document the previous incidents in case of a lawsuit.

54. **(c)** The nurse manager would make the decision whether the hospital rules should be broken in this case.

55. **(a)** The proper chain of command would require you to notify the patient's nurse of the critical value first. He or she may ask you to page the resident or call the doctor. (If the patient's resident or doctor is on the nursing unit, you may notify him or her and then notify the nurse.)

NOTES

56. There is a court order on a pediatric patient's chart prohibiting the parents from leaving the nursing unit with their child. You see the parents walking toward the elevator with the child. You would:
    a. call security
    b. find the patient's nurse
    c. try to stop the parents from getting on the elevator
    d. call the nurse manager

57. A patient admitted with a diagnosis of metastatic carcinoma would be assigned to which of the following units?
    a. orthopedics
    b. neurology
    c. oncology
    d. telemetry

58. A patient experiencing arrhythmia would likely be admitted to which of the following units?
    a. TICU
    b. pulmonary
    c. neurology
    d. telemetry

59. A patient admitted post-MVA from ER would likely be admitted to which of the following units?
    a. CICU
    b. TICU
    c. urology
    d. MICU

60. A patient with a diagnosis of CHF would be admitted to which of the following units?
    a. pediatrics
    b. MICU
    c. CICU
    d. orthopedics

61. A doctor's order is written for a consent to be prepared for a CABG. You would write out the consent to read:
    a. capillary and arterial bilateral graft
    b. corneal anterior bilateral graft
    c. coronary artery bypass graft
    d. contrast anterior balloon graph

62. Which of the following specimens would need to be placed in a bag of crushed ice immediately?
    a. arterial blood
    b. stool
    c. venous blood
    d. sterile urine

63. A patient admitted with the following diagnosis would be placed in respiratory isolation:
    a. AIDS
    b. RA
    c. TB
    d. COPD

64. A patient with Parkinson's disease would be admitted to which of the following units?
    a. neurology
    b. orthopedics
    c. pulmonary
    d. surgical

65. A child is admitted to PICU with injuries that do not seem realistic given the parents' explanation. Which of the following agencies would be called in to investigate the cause of the injuries?
    a. APS
    b. OSHA
    c. CPS
    d. DPS

☑ ANSWERS AND RATIONALE

56. **(a)** Call security immediately.

57. **(c)** A patient with a diagnosis of metastatic carcinoma would be admitted to the oncology unit.

58. **(d)** A patient experiencing arrhythmia (a deviation from the normal pattern of the heartbeat) would be admitted to the telemetry unit.

59. **(b)** A patient admitted after an MVA (motor vehicle accident) would likely be admitted to TICU (trauma intensive care unit) from the ER (emergency room).

60. **(c)** A patient with a diagnosis of CHF (congestive heart failure) would be admitted to CICU (coronary intensive care unit); also may be called CVICU (cardiovascular intensive care unit).

61. **(c)** CABG is the abbreviation for coronary artery bypass graft.

62. **(a)** Arterial blood samples must be placed on ice immediately after being drawn.

63. **(c)** A patient admitted with TB (tuberculosis) would be placed in isolation to prevent transmission of disease by contact or droplet. A patient admitted with a diagnosis of AIDS (acquired immunodeficiency syndrome) would not be placed in respiratory isolation, because universal precautions are used with all patients' body fluids and AIDS is not transmitted by droplet. RA is rheumatoid arthritis and COPD is chronic obstructive pulmonary disease; neither requires any type of isolation.

Droplet infection is the invasion of a pathogenic agent conveyed by particles, as when carried in a spray from the nose or mouth.

64. **(a)** A patient with a diagnosis of Parkinson's disease would be admitted to the neurology unit.

65. **(c)** CPS (Child Protective Services) would investigate possible child abuse. Health care workers are required by law to report suspected child abuse. One indication is when the parent's explanations of the injuries do not match the type of injuries sustained by the child.

APS—Adult Protective services
OSHA—Occupational Safety and Health Administration
DPS—Department of Public Safety

TEST-TAKING TIP

Prepare yourself mentally for the exam. Try positive mental imagery. Imagine yourself taking the test with the confidence that you are selecting the correct answers. Imagine yourself receiving a passing score. Having positive thoughts about your ability to perform can affect your actual performance.

66. A patient is concerned about her insurance paying for hospitalization and what her options are when she is discharged. Which of the following hospital department personnel would assist her with these concerns:
    a. case management
    b. risk management
    c. infection control
    d. quality management

67. HIPAA regulations require that patients be given the following when admitted to the hospital:
    a. advance directives
    b. a form indicating if they want to be listed in the hospital directory
    c. a form indicating choice of meals
    d. blood transfusion consent or refusal

☑ ANSWERS AND RATIONALE

66. **(a)** Case management personnel act as a liaison between patient, doctor, and the insurance company.

67. **(b)** A form indicating if they want to be listed in the hospital directory. HIPAA provides regulations to protect patient information.

TEST-TAKING TIP

Get plenty of rest the night before the exam.

The Certification Review Exam: Breakdown of Content and Mock Examination

The following mock exam contains questions representative of those you will see on the certification exam sponsored by the National Association of Health Unit Coordinators. Taking this exam will assist you in assessing your knowledge base and preparedness for taking the actual national exam. The answer for each question is provided on the page that follows. Page numbers for the textbook, *Health Unit Coordinating*, 5th edition, are provided for more detailed information regarding answers to the questions that have specific answers. This exam, like Chapter 24 and the national exam, addresses work-related situations requiring communication, critical thinking, and problem-solving skills. There may be more than one answer to these questions that could apply, and one that would be the best answer for the given situation. Chapter numbers for the textbook are provided in the answer section when the entire chapter supplies a foundation of knowledge, including communication and problem-solving techniques, that would be helpful in answering a specific question.

Breakdown of Exam Content
The following breakdown applies to both the National Certification Exam and the Mock Exam presented here.

48% Coordination of the Unit
A. Operations
    1. Supplies and services management
    2. Information management—patient record, unit, staff organization
B. Communication
    1. Equipment
    2. Skills
C. Orientation and training personnel
D. Safety

10% Confidentiality and Patient Rights

6% Critical Thinking
A. Problem identification and resources
B. Prioritization and decision making

31% Order Transcription
A. Process
B. Classifications, diagnostic, dietary, nursing, pharmacy, treatment, miscellaneous
C. Medical terms, abbreviations, and symbols

5% Professional Development

Health Unit Coordinator
Mock Certification Exam

1. A discrepancy report sent by the central service department is a list of items:
   a. Used from a nursing unit supply closet that were not charged to any patient
   b. Not used from the nursing unit supply closet
   c. Found in the nursing unit supply closet that do not belong there
   d. Charged to the wrong patient

2. Which of the following items cannot be sent in the pneumatic tube system?
   a. An empty chart binder
   b. Patient chart forms
   c. Central supply items
   d. Cerebral spinal fluid

3. The printer in the nursing station is not functioning properly. The health unit coordinator would notify the:
   a. Director of nurses
   b. Computer training instructor
   c. Hospital information systems department
   d. Maintenance department

4. An inpatient is a patient who is admitted to the hospital for longer than:
   a. 12 hours
   b. 24 hours
   c. 1 hour
   d. 48 hours

5. An IV infusion pump has been discontinued on a patient. It would be stored in the:
   a. Dirty utility room
   b. Patient's room
   c. Hallway
   d. Clean utility room

6. A package of stoma bags that were not used is found in a discharged patient's room. The health unit coordinator would complete a/an:
   a. Insurance request slip
   b. Charge requisition
   c. Credit slip for the central service department
   d. Envelope to mail to patient

7. The health unit coordinator notes that there are four labeled chart forms in a discharged patient's chart that have no documentation on them. She or he would:
   a. Place the forms in the waste basket
   b. Send the forms to health records in case they are needed
   c. Place the forms in another patient's chart with the new patient's label over the discharged patient's label
   d. Shred the forms

8. You have been asked to thin a patient's chart. The thinned-out records would be:
   a. Sent to health records immediately
   b. Placed in an envelope, labeled with patient's ID labels, and kept on the nursing unit until the patient is discharged or moved
   c. Placed in a second chart labeled with patient ID labels and labeled as chart # 2
   d. Shredded

9. *Patient-centered care* is care that involves:
   a. A registered nurse that will have total responsibility for a patient
   b. All departments that deal with the patient using a multidisciplinary approach
   c. Only the nursing department
   d. A group of specialists that focus on specific diseases

☑ *ANSWERS AND RATIONALE*

1. **(a)** Used from a nursing unit supply closet that were not charged to any patient. p. 98

2. **(d)** Cerebral spinal fluid (CSF) specimens obtained by a painful procedure cannot be sent in the pneumatic tube system. The system may beak down, the specimen may be misdirected or the tubes may leak or break. pp. 243, 488

3. **(c)** Hospital information systems would be responsible for repairing electronic equipment. p. 23

4. **(b)** 24 hours. p. 15

5. **(a)** The IV infusion pump would be stored in the dirty utility room until picked up by a central supply technician to be sterilized. p. 97

6. **(c)** The stoma bags would be credited to the patient's bill by completing a credit slip for the central service department. p. 98

7. **(d)** Forms that do not have documentation on them and that contain patient ID labels are shredded for patient confidentiality. p. 48

8. **(b)** Placed in an envelope, labeled with patient's ID label, and kept on the nursing unit until the patient is transferred of discharged. You would also write the date thinned and initial the envelope. p. 155

9. **(b)** Patient-centered care is care that involves all departments dealing with the patient in a multidisciplinary approach. It may also be called *patient-focused care*. p. 36

NOTES

10. Security of patient information laws, including a patient's right to not have his or her name listed in the hospital directory, are specified in the:
    a. Americans with Disability Act (ADA)
    b. Occupational Safety and Health Act (OSHA)
    c. Health Insurance Portability and Accountability Act (HIPAA)
    d. Fair Labor Standard Act (FLSA)

11. A health unit coordinator with over 20 years of experience is hired for a busy orthopedic unit. He has good organizational skills and immediately notices that the nursing station is set up in a way that makes the health unit coordinator's job difficult. He should:
    a. Make the changes that would better organize the unit
    b. Discuss the changes with his coworkers on his shift
    c. Discuss the changes with the nurse manager
    d. Discuss the changes with the other health unit coordinators

12. Which of the following would be important for the health unit coordinator to note on the patient census work sheet kept near the telephone:
    a. A patient is scheduled for a CBC
    b. A patient is on a temporary pass
    c. A patient is scheduled for a chest x-ray
    d. A patient is Catholic

13. A nurse on another unit has called your unit three times regarding transferring a patient from her unit to the unit where you are working. The nurse who will be caring for the patient to be transferred states that she is too busy to receive another patient now. The nurse from the other unit becomes abusive to you, stating that she is just as busy and would like to bring the patient now. You would:
    a. Tell the nurse on the telephone not to kill the messenger
    b. Tell the nurse on the telephone to just go ahead and send the patient
    c. Inform the nurse that will be receiving the patient to fight her own fights
    d. Ask the nurse to hold while you obtain a definite time when she will be able to send the patient

14. You witness a coworker copying a patient's records that she knows personally to take home. You would:
    a. Mind your business
    b. Advise him that if he takes the records, you will report the incident to the nurse manager
    c. Call security immediately
    d. Notify the nurse manager

15. Which of the following departments would intervene if a patient had concerns regarding his or her insurance not paying for his or her hospital stay?
    a. Case management
    b. Risk management
    c. Quality assurance
    d. Medical assistant

16. When leaving the nursing station to take a lunch break, you should:
    a. Turn the computer off
    b. Sign off so that your ID number will not be used
    c. Leave the computer with your sign-on so others can use it
    d. Ask one of the nurses to monitor the computer in your absence

✓ *ANSWERS AND RATIONALE*

10. **(c)** The Health Insurance Portability and Accountability Act (HIPAA) includes laws that protect patient information. Releasing patient information without permission is not only a violation of ethics but also illegal. p. 83

11. **(c)** Any changes to the organization of the nursing unit should be discussed with the nurse manager. p. 105

12. **(b)** Patient is on a temporary pass. p. 100

13. **(d)** Ask the nurse to hold while you obtain a definite time when she will be able to send the patient. (Chapter 5 addresses telephone etiquette and assertiveness)

14. **(d)** Notify the nurse manager. The coworker is committing an unlawful act. pp. 83, 84

15. **(a)** A case manager acts as a liaison among the patient, doctor, and insurance company. p. 22

16. **(b)** Sign off so that others cannot use your ID code. p. 49

NOTES

17. Which of the following actions could cause a *serious* error when using the fax machine?
    a. Placing the papers to be faxed in the machine upside down
    b. Automatically using the redial button to fax pharmacy copies
    c. Dialing the number each time you want to fax
    d. Using the fax machine to make copies

18. E-mails sent by you or to you at work:
    a. Are protected by confidentiality laws
    b. Are never monitored
    c. May be monitored
    d. Are always monitored

19. Your computer activity on the Internet:
    a. Cannot be tracked
    b. Is protected by confidentiality laws
    c. Is constantly tracked
    d. May be tracked

20. A patient approaches the nursing station to tell you that his roommate is smoking in their bathroom and the smell bothers him. You would:
    a. Advise him that he could be moved to another room
    b. Suggest that he could use the bathroom in the hall
    c. Tell him that you will notify their nurse
    d. Call security immediately

21. A nurse who works on the same unit as you do continuously makes insulting remarks to you, such as, "you're just a unit clerk." or "you had to go to school to do this?" Your best response would be:
    a. Ignore her and hope she will get the message
    b. Tell the nurse manager that the nurse is constantly being rude to you
    c. Ask her to just talk to you when it concerns work
    d. Tell her that it hurts your feelings when she downgrades your position

22. A nurse aggressively tells you that you forgot to notify him about a personal phone call. You answered the call when the nurse was in the middle of a conversation and meant to tell him when he was finished, but forgot. Your best response would be:
    a. Tell him that he shouldn't get so many personal calls anyway
    b. Tell him he was busy at the time and you forgot to tell him
    c. Tell him you're not his personal secretary
    d. Ignore his comments

23. A patient's wife confides in you that they have no food in the house and can't afford the medications that her husband needs. The doctor has written a discharge order for the next day. What should you do?
    a. Notify the social services department
    b. Notify risk management
    c. Advise her to call the welfare department
    d. Tell her you are sorry to hear of her difficulties

24. A respiratory therapist asks you to make a new identification bracelet for 121 bed 1. You would:
    a. Make the identification bracelet
    b. Ask for the patient's name
    c. Tell him to make it himself
    d. Refuse to make the bracelet

25. A Native American patient approaches the nursing station and tells you that neither his doctor nor his nurse understand his culture and he feels disrespected when he tries to talk to them. Your best response would be:
    a. Ask for more information and advise him that you will relay his concerns to his nurse
    b. Tell him that we all come from different cultures and he can't expect everyone to be aware of everyone's cultural differences
    c. Advise him to keep trying to talk to his doctor and nurse
    d. Call the nurse manager to talk to him

✔ ANSWERS AND RATIONALE

17. **(b)** Using the redial button without checking the number to which your document is being sent could send the document to the wrong location. This could cause a breach of confidentiality. p. 48

18. **(c)** Your e-mails may be monitored. pp. 49, 50

19. **(d)** Computer activity, including using the internet and looking up lab results of a personal friend on another unit, may be tracked. pp. 49, 50

20. **(c)** Tell him that you will notify his nurse. (Chapter 5 addresses Maslow's Hierarchy of Needs and telecommunications skills)

21. **(d)** Tell her that it hurts your feelings when she downgrades your position. (Chapter 5 addresses communication and assertiveness skills)

22. **(b)** Tell him he was busy at the time and you forgot to tell him. Accept responsibility for your error without beating yourself up. p. 70

23. **(a)** Notify the social services department. You would also notify the patient's nurse. p. 354

24. **(b)** Ask for the patient's name. Patients should be referred to by their name, not their room and bed number or their diagnosis p. 60

25. **(a)** Ask for more information and advise him that you will relay his concerns to his nurse. It is important to provide culturally sensitive care. p. 65

NOTES

26. A patient is admitted in critical condition to the intensive care unit. A group of her concerned family members are standing in the hall. The noise level is getting very loud and is disturbing other patients. You would:
    a. Show them to the waiting area and advise them that you will let the nurse know where they are waiting
    b. Ask them to keep the noise down because they are bothering the other patients
    c. Do nothing, they have enough problems
    d. Call security to talk to them

27. A wife of an elderly patient angrily complains to you that her husband has been lying in a wet bed for two hours. Which of the following responses would most likely be interpreted as aggressive?
    a. "I can see that you are angry. I will tell his nurse that he needs attention immediately."
    b. "You told me just five minutes ago and I told his nurse. What else can I do?"
    c. "I will ask his nurse to come to his room as soon as possible."
    d. "Jane said she will be in his room in just another five minutes."

28. A patient continually stops by the nursing station to talk to you. She told you that she is widowed and has not seen any of her children in the three days that she has been in the hospital. What need is she expressing?
    a. Self actualization
    b. Physical
    c. Self esteem
    d. Love and belonging

29. It is an extremely busy day and you are in the middle of transcribing orders on a post-op patient. Dr. Jones arrives on the nursing unit and insists that you stop what you are doing to get him a cup of coffee. An assertive response would be:
    a. "I'm not here to be a waitress!"
    b. "You can get your own coffee!"
    c. "Ok, I will quick get your coffee and finish these orders when I return."
    d. "I'm really busy right now—the coffee is in the report room."

30. Dr. Smith's handwriting is very difficult to read. Often you have to take the chart to the patient's nurse to assist you in reading his orders and still end up having to call him for verification. The best solution for this problem would be:
    a. Ask Dr. Smith to print his orders
    b. Ask the hospital CEO to talk to him about his handwriting
    c. Ask Dr. Smith to wait until you read his orders before leaving in case you have questions
    d. Report him to the nurse manager and ask her to talk to him about his handwriting

31. Dr. Norman makes rounds at 0700 every morning because she has a busy surgery schedule. She is constantly irritated because it takes time to locate her charts and her patients' daily lab results. The best solution for this problem would be:
    a. When you arrive to work, print all of the daily lab results on Dr. Norman's patients; place them on the front of their charts, and stack all of her patient's charts on a cart.
    b. When Dr. Norman arrives on the unit, ignore all other tasks and assist her in finding her patients' lab results and charts
    c. Ask the nurse manager for additional help for that hour or so that Dr. Norman is making her rounds
    d. Ignore her irritability. She is being unreasonable, so let her find her patients' charts and lab results herself.

✔ *ANSWERS AND RATIONALE*

26. **(a)** Show them to the waiting area and advise them that you will let the nurse know where they are waiting. Point out to them that they will be more comfortable in the waiting area, and you could suggest that they go to the cafeteria for coffee or a bite to eat. p. 59

27. **(b)** "You told me just five minutes ago and I told his nurse. What else can I do?" That response is very aggressive. Starting the sentence with "You" places the other person on the defensive. Any of the other responses would be appropriate. p. 66

28. **(d)** Love and belonging. pp. 59, 60

29. **(d)** "I'm really busy right now—the coffee is in the report room." would be an assertive response. It is not your responsibility to bring coffee to the doctors. Responses *a* and *b* would be aggressive and *c* would be nonassertive. p. 67

30. **(c)** Ask Dr Smith to wait until you read his orders before leaving in case you have questions. Doctors usually appreciate this and it will save you and the doctor time. p. 172

31. **(a)** When you arrive to work, print all of the daily lab results on Dr. Norman's patients and place them on the front of their charts, and tack all of her patients' charts on a cart. This will save Dr. Norman time and will save you from constant interruptions and dealing with her irritability while she is making rounds. (Chapter 7 addresses problem-solving skills; see also pp. 106, 107)

NOTES

32. You have floated to NICU and you have never worked there before. One of the nurses who is routinely assigned to that unit tells you that you are incompetent and don't know what you are doing when you can't find forms she asked you to find. Your best response would be:
    a. "I'm sorry, I guess I am incompetent."
    b. "Why don't you find them yourself? You work here all the time!"
    c. Ignore her and call another health unit coordinator to assist you in finding the forms
    d. "It must seem that I'm incompetent. I have not worked on this unit before. Can you tell me where those forms are stored?"

33. Dr. Williams asks you how her patient, Manny Gomez is doing. Your best response would be:
    a. "I'm not a nurse; you will need to speak to his nurse."
    b. "I don't know; I'm the health unit coordinator."
    c. "I will find Mr. Gomez's nurse, Sue, for you."
    d. "I guess he's fine. I haven't heard any different."

34. Dr. Cohen throws a report in front of you and tells you that it was filed in the wrong patient's chart. Your best response would be:
    a. "I haven't even been here for the last two days. I didn't do it."
    b. "Pat did all the filing for me today. Talk to her."
    c. "I can see that you're upset. I'll file it in the correct patient's chart. Please don't throw misfiled reports at me again."
    d. "You don't have to be so rude!"

35. A student health unit coordinator is placed on your nursing unit. You have worked with her for a week and notice that she is not retaining anything you have told her. She takes longer breaks than she should and becomes defensive when you show her what she is doing wrong. The best response would be to:
    a. Keep quiet about it. She will only be there for a short time.
    b. Tell all the other health unit coordinators that she is incompetent and to double check her work if they work with her
    c. Refuse to train her anymore without an explanation
    d. Talk to the student's instructor and the nurse manager

36. You are a new employee and have been placed with an experienced health unit coordinator for two weeks of orientation. The health unit coordinator continuously leaves you alone and is not spending time to orient you to the nursing unit. You feel she is taking advantage of you. Your best action would be to:
    a. Report the health unit coordinator to the nurse manager
    b. Look for another job
    c. Tell the health unit coordinator how you feel and ask her to spend some time showing you what you need to know
    d. Ask the nurses on the unit to assist you in the health unit coordinator's absence

37. You notice a student nurse sitting in the employee lounge crying. She tells you that she helped a patient to the bathroom and then found out that he was on complete bed rest. Your best action would be to:
    a. Advise her to page her instructor immediately
    b. Report her to the nurse manager
    c. Place a call to the patient's doctor to report the incident
    d. Tell her to keep quiet if there was no apparent harm done

32. **(d)** "It must seem that I'm incompetent. I have not worked on this unit before. Can you tell me where those forms are stored?" This response is recognizing that there is some validity to the nurse's comment, but you are not internalizing the comment. p. 70

33. **(c)** "I will find Mr. Gomez's nurse, Sue, for you." This response is demonstrating your willingness to be helpful. pp. 64, 65

34. **(c)** "I can see that you're upset. I'll file it in the correct patient's chart. Please don't throw misfiled reports at me again." p. 67

35. **(d)** Talk to the student's instructor and the nurse manager. You would not be doing the student, the hospital, or the instructor justice by not bringing it to their attention. p. 82

36. **(c)** Tell the health unit coordinator how you feel and ask her to spend some time showing you what you need to know. p. 67

37. **(a)** Advise her to page her instructor immediately. p. 82

NOTES

38. National guidelines serving as a model of performance by which health unit coordinators shall conduct their actions are known as a:
    a. Standard of Practice
    b. Code of Ethics
    c. Job description
    d. Policy

39. A newly hired nurse has been assigned to observe with you for a day. He acts bored and resentful while you are demonstrating use of the computer. You would:
    a. Tell him to read a book or something if he is bored; it wasn't your idea to have him sit with you
    b. Ignore him and do your job as usual; it's easier to do your job without explaining what you are doing to someone who doesn't want to know anyway
    c. Report him to the nurse manager and ask that he be placed with someone else
    d. Remind him that there are times when the health unit coordinator will be away from the desk and he will want to locate lab results or order a stat lab

40. When a copy of a patient's current records is requested in a doctor's order and you are not sure of the proper procedure, you would:
    a. Follow the procedure for copying patient records as outlined in the policy and procedure manual
    b. Ask a health unit coordinator on another unit
    c. Ask one of the nurses
    d. Call the doctor and ask his or her preference

41. Which of the following tasks would be outside the health unit coordinator's scope of practice?
    a. Ordering supplies and equipment as required
    b. Answering all visitor questions relating to patient care, treatment, and progress
    c. Transcribing written doctor's orders for patients' diagnostic tests and treatments
    d. Communicating all new doctor's orders to the patient's nurses

42. A D.O. (doctor of osteopathy) places special emphasis on the relationship of organs with the:
    a. Nervous system
    b. Musculoskeletal system
    c. Endocrine system
    d. Pituitary gland

43. HMO is an abbreviation meaning:
    a. Homeopathic doctor
    b. Heart-monitored operation
    c. Hormone maintenance organ
    d. Health Maintenance Organization

44. The day set aside to celebrate National Health Unit Coordinator Day is:
    a. July 7
    b. January 20
    c. September 9
    d. August 23

45. An effective method of preparing for your yearly evaluation would be to:
    a. Start a petition listing your best qualities and have coworkers sign it
    b. Ask doctors and nurses with whom you have a good relationship to write letters of recommendation
    c. Work all the overtime you possibly can and do extra favors for your nurse manager
    d. Keep a diary of in-services, educational classes, professional association involvement, and any extra contributions that you have made in your work to take with you to your evaluation

46. A fire has been reported and the fire code announced. Your next action would be to:
    a. Start evacuating all the patients
    b. Gather all the patient charts for removal
    c. Do nothing until instructed to act
    d. Close all the patient room doors

☑ **ANSWERS AND RATIONALE**

38. **(a)** Standard of Practice is used as a model of performance by which health unit coordinators shall conduct their actions. p. 88

39. **(d)** Remind him that there are times when the health unit coordinator will be away from the desk and he will want to locate lab results or order a stat lab. p. 67

40. **(a)** Follow the procedure for copying patient records as outlined in the policy and procedure manual. p. 84

41. **(b)** Answering all visitor questions relating to patient care, treatment, and progress. pp. 7–10

42. **(b)** Musculoskeletal system. Structural problems are corrected by manipulation. p. 18

43. **(d)** Health Maintenance Organization. p. 24

44. **(d)** August 23. The date represents the first meeting to establish the National Association of Health Unit Coordinators held in Phoenix, Arizona, in 1983. p. 5

45. **(d)** Keep a diary of in-services, educational classes, professional association involvement, and any extra contributions that you have made in your work to take with you to your evaluation. p. 86

46. **(d)** Close all the patient room doors. p. 434

NOTES

47. When a patient code arrest is occurring on the unit where you are working, your responsibility would be:
    a. Over once the code is called; the code team takes over
    b. To go to the intensive care unit and arrange a bed placement for the patient
    c. To call all of the patient's family to come to the hospital
    d. To remain on the unit and carry out orders as given to you

48. It is not necessary to isolate a patient with HIV because:
    a. HIV is not at all contagious
    b. Universal or Standard Precautions are used with all patients
    c. All health care workers are vaccinated to protect them from HIV
    d. Patients with HIV are given medication that makes it impossible for them to transmit the disease to someone else

49. The abbreviation PPE stands for:
    a. Personal protective equipment
    b. Pre-prepared equipment
    c. Post-protective exception
    d. Privately prepared equipment

50. The best protection from infection is:
    a. One-a-Day vitamins
    b. Frequent doctor visits
    c. Good handwashing habits
    d. Staying out of patient rooms

51. An example of a situation in which the hospital would institute a disaster procedure would be:
    a. An airplane crash
    b. 10% of health care workers employed at hospital falling ill
    c. Two patients coding at the same time
    d. Three patients being brought into ER from a car accident

52. Infectious diseases are usually not transmitted by:
    a. Air
    b. Droplet
    c. Personal contact
    d. Inanimate objects

53. Which of the following is a common hospital-acquired infection?
    a. Staphylococcus
    b. Mononucleosis
    c. Coccidioidomycosis
    d. Pneumonitis

54. A condition transmitted by body fluids that is more contagious than AIDS is:
    a. PID
    b. HBV
    c. URI
    d. UTI

55. A well-dressed man approaches the nurse's station and tells you that he is the attorney representing Mr. Ross Engelhart, who has *NINP* written on his chart (at his request). The man asks if Mr. Engelhart is a patient on our unit. Your best response would be to:
    a. Deny having any knowledge of a Mr. Engelhart
    b. Tell him the Mr. Engelhart's room number
    c. Call security
    d. Ask the man to wait while you ask Mr. Engelhart if he is really his attorney

56. A friend of yours is a patient on the unit where you work. Her husband is also your friend. She and her husband are having marital problems. The husband has visited his wife once since her hospitalization, but calls you at home to ask why his wife is in the hospital. Your best response would be:
    a. Answer his question because he is still her husband and is really concerned
    b. Advise him that you can not discuss his wife's hospitalization with him
    c. Tell him to mind his own business; if his wife wanted him to know, she would have told him.
    d. Give him his wife's room telephone number and tell him to call her

☑ ANSWERS AND RATIONALE

47. **(d)** Remain on the unit and carry out orders as given to you. pp. 434, 435
48. **(b)** Universal or Standard Precautions are used with all patients. p. 431
49. **(a)** Personal protective equipment that includes goggles, gloves, masks, and so on. p. 432
50. **(c)** The best protection from infection is to develop good hand washing habits. p. 432
51. **(a)** An airplane crash is an example of a disaster that could involve multiple patients. p. 434
52. **(d)** Infectious diseases are usually not transmitted by inanimate objects. pp. 430–432
53. **(a)** Staphylococcus is a common hospital-acquired or nosocomial infection. p. 433
54. **(b)** HBV (hepatitis B virus) is a condition transmitted by body fluids that is more contagious than AIDS (acquired immune deficiency syndrome). p. 433
55. **(a)** Deny having any knowledge of a Mr. Engelhart. If the man persists, refer him to the nurse manager. pp. 83, 84
56. **(b)** Advise him that you cannot discuss his wife's hospitalization with him. pp. 83, 84

NOTES

57. A patient admitted to the nursing unit where you work asks you to show him his chart. Your best response would be:
    a. Tell him patients are not allowed to see their charts
    b. Advise him that you will notify his nurse and/or doctor of his request
    c. Allow him to look at his chart
    d. Show him only the doctor's progress notes

58. There is a court order prohibiting the father of a pediatric patient from having any contact with the child or his mother. You see the father step off the elevator and walk toward the patient's room. Your best response would be to:
    a. Call security immediately
    b. Walk over to him and tell him to leave the hospital
    c. Do nothing; maybe they can work out their problems if left alone
    d. Call the nurse manager

59. An informed consent means that:
    a. The surgery department has been informed of the patient's signature on the surgical consent
    b. The surgeon has written the exact procedure on the patient's order sheet
    c. The consent form has been prepared and the nurse has been informed that it is ready to be signed
    d. The surgical procedure, risks, alternatives, and expected outcome have been explained to the patient

60. The Joint Commission on Accreditation of Health Care Organizations requires that all hospitals provide a copy of the following to patients upon admission:
    a. A list of any violations found during the hospital inspection by JCAHO
    b. A list of all doctors that will be involved with the patient's care
    c. A copy of the patient's bill of rights
    d. A copy of the hospital's accreditation

61. A patient approaches the nurse's station and tells you that he is very unhappy with the care and his doctor's treatment. He tells you that he is leaving the hospital. Your best response would be:
    a. Ask him to please wait until you ask his nurse to come talk to him
    b. Advise him that he cannot leave until his doctor writes the order
    c. Tell him you will call security
    d. Tell him that it is decision and ask him to sign the leaving against medical advice form

62. A friend of yours is admitted to the hospital with a diagnosis of pneumonia. He has confided in you that he thinks he may have AIDS. You would share this information with:
    a. Your friend's doctor
    b. The nurse caring for him
    c. The case manager assigned to him
    d. No one

63. A nurse from another unit approaches you in the cafeteria and tells you that she heard there was a patient admitted to the unit where you work who was involved in a shooting that morning. Your best response would be:
    a. Tell her, as she is a nurse and would have access to information anyway
    b. Just tell her yes but provide no details
    c. Tell her to ask someone else because you don't want to get in any trouble
    d. Remind her that you can't discuss patient information

64. A patient approaches the nurse's station and tells you that she is having second thoughts about a procedure she is to have that morning. Your best response would be to:
    a. Tell her that everyone has second thoughts and it will work out fine
    b. Advise her that it is a little late to be having second thoughts, because the procedure has already been ordered
    c. Tell her that she signed the consent and that the time to voice doubt has passed
    d. Tell her you will ask her nurse to come in and discuss it with her

☑ *ANSWERS AND RATIONALE*

57. **(b)** Advise him that you will notify his nurse and/or doctor of his request. p. 84

58. **(a)** Call security immediately. p. 86

59. **(d)** The surgical procedure, risks, alternatives, and expected outcome have been explained to the patient. p 89

60. **(c)** A copy of the patient's bill of rights is provided to each patient upon admission. p. 87

61. **(a)** Ask him to please wait until you ask his nurse to come talk to him. pp. 402, 403

62. **(d)** You would share this information with no one. p. 83

63. **(d)** Remind her that you can't discuss patient information. pp. 83, 84

64. **(d)** Tell her you will ask her nurse to come in and discuss it with her. (Chapter 5 addresses Maslow's Hierarchy of Needs and communication skills, and Chapter 6 addresses informed consent)

NOTES

65. A patient's relative passes the nurses' station and stops to ask you if you know how much weight her sister has lost since admission. Your best response would be:
    a. Tell her that you don't have access to that information even though you do
    b. Look it up as she is the patient's sister and is just concerned
    c. Tell her not to ask questions that you can't answer
    d. Advise her that you cannot discuss patient information

66. A patient tells you that her doctor talks over her head and she is concerned about her condition. She tells you that the doctor stops in her room to tell her the test results and then leaves without asking if she understands what they mean. Your best response would be:
    a. Tell her that you know what she means; doctors are like that
    b. Just listen and don't make any comments that could get you in trouble
    c. Tell her to demand that he talk to her
    d. Advise her that you will relay her concerns to her nurse and will ask her nurse to come talk to her

67. A consult with Dr. John Silverman has been ordered for a patient admitted to the orthopedic unit with a fractured femur. When looking in the doctor roster for Dr. Silverman's telephone number, you find two Dr. John Silvermans listed. You would:
    a. Call the ordering doctor to determine which doctor he wanted to consult
    b. Call the Dr. John Silverman that is the orthopedist
    c. Ask the patient if she knows which doctor was to do the consult
    d. Ask the patient's nurse if he knows which Dr. Silverman is to do the consult

68. You are working in the surgical intensive care unit. A consulting specialist writes an order that a patient may be transferred to a floor unit. You would:
    a. Call the attending doctor to obtain an order to transfer the patient
    b. Transfer the patient according to the consulting specialist's order
    c. Wait until the attending doctor comes in to see the patient
    d. Ask the nurse manager what to do

69. A doctor wrote orders on a patient but forgot to sign them. Hospital policy states that orders cannot be carried out until signed. You would:
    a. Ask a nurse to sign them even though she doesn't know the doctor who wrote them
    b. Sign the doctor's name and ask him to write his signature when he makes rounds in the morning
    c. Place a call to the doctor and advise the patient's nurse so she can take the telephone orders
    d. Leave the orders until someone signs them

70. You observe a man becoming increasingly angry as he is speaking to a nurse on the unit where you are working. You can see that she is becoming anxious. You would:
    a. Walk over and advise the visitor to calm down
    b. Ignore the situation; it is probably your imagination
    c. Call security
    d. Call the nurse manager

☑ *ANSWERS AND RATIONALE*

65. **(d)** Advise her that you cannot discuss patient information. pp. 83, 84

66. **(d)** Advise her that you will relay her concerns to her nurse and will ask her nurse to come talk to her. (Chapter 5 addresses Maslow's Hierarchy of Needs and communication skills)

67. **(b)** Call the Dr. John Silverman that is the orthopedist. p. 47

68. **(a)** Call the attending doctor to obtain an order to transfer the patient. pp. 14, 18

69. **(c)** Place a call to the doctor and advise that patient's nurse so she can take the telephone orders. p. 46

70. **(c)** Call security immediately. p. 86

NOTES

71. A nurse asks you to call a code, a doctor is waiting for you to assist him in locating a patient's chart, a visitor is standing at the desk to ask a question, and the telephone is ringing. In what sequence would you handle the tasks?
    a. (1) Call the code, (2) answer the telephone, (3) answer the visitor's question, and (4) assist the doctor in finding his patient's chart
    b. (1) Answer the visitor's question (visitors always have priority), (2) call the code, (3) answer the telephone, and (4) assist the doctor in finding his patient's chart
    c. (1) Assist the doctor in finding his patient's chart (doctors always come first), (2) call the code, (3) answer the phone, and (4) answer the visitor's question
    d. (1) Answer the telephone (the telephone always takes priority), (2) call the code, (3) assist the doctor in finding his patient's chart, and (4) answer the visitor's question

72. You answer the nursing unit telephone and a patient's husband asks you in a loud voice: "What the *#$% is going on in that place? I have called four times today to speak to the nurse that's supposed to be taking care of my wife and she has never called me back!" His tone is becoming angrier and louder as he continues. Your best response would be:
    a. Hang up the telephone; you do not need to listen to such abusive language
    b. Tell him to calm down using the same angry tone of voice that he is using
    c. Ask him to hold while you find his nurse
    d. Tell him you feel he is becoming abusive and to please call back in a few minutes so you can talk about the situation calmly

73. When transcribing a patient's orders, you note that the hospitalist has ordered ampicillin on Mary Jackson. Her chart is labeled that she is allergic to penicillin. You would:
    a. Notify the hospitalist of the patient's allergy to penicillin
    b. Ask the patient if she is really allergic to penicillin
    c. Transcribe the order as written as the hospitalist certainly saw the allergy indicated on the chart
    d. Ask the patient how severe her allergy is and if she has ever taken ampicillin

74. It is 2:00 PM and you discover an order written for a patient that reads, "PCXR this am" that you didn't see earlier. You would:
    a. Order the PCXR stat
    b. Call the doctor that wrote the order to ask what to do
    c. Ask the patient's nurse what to do
    d. Order the PCXR, call the diagnostic imaging department to explain the situation, and notify the patient's nurse

75. A symbol or computer order number is written above an order on the physician's order sheet:
    a. Prior to completing that step of transcription, to indicate that you have read the order
    b. After completing that step of transcription to indicate that you have completed that step
    c. After you have completed transcribing the entire set of doctor's orders
    d. Never

76. Which of the following orders is a *standing order?*
    a. Demerol 75 mg IM q 4 hr for severe pain
    b. CBC this am
    c. Valium 10 mg PO on call to cath lab
    d. Regular diet

77. Which of the following orders is a *standing PRN order?*
    a. Demerol 100 mg IM in am prior to colonoscopy
    b. PT q am × 3 days
    c. Tylenol 500 mg PO q 4–6 hr for H/A
    d. Synthroid 0.05 mg PO q am

✔ *ANSWERS AND RATIONALE*

71. **(a)** (1) Call the code, (2) answer the telephone, (3) answer the visitor's question, and (4) assist the doctor in finding his patient's chart. You can acknowledge the presence of the doctor and visitor to let them know that you will be with them shortly while placing the call for the code and answering the ringing telephone. pp. 102, 103

72. **(d)** Tell him you feel he is becoming abusive and to please call back in a few minutes so you can talk about the situation calmly. p. 71

73. **(a)** Notify the hospitalist of the patient's allergy to penicillin. pp. 117, 130

74. **(d)** Order the PCXR (portable chest x-ray), call the diagnostic imaging department to explain the situation, and notify the patient's nurse. (Chapter 7 addresses problem-solving skills; see also pp. 106, 107)

75. **(b)** After completing that step of transcription, to indicate that you have completed that step. p. 166

76. **(d)** An order for a regular diet would stay in effect until the doctor changes or discontinues the order, and would therefore be a standing order. p. 163

77. **(c)** Tylenol 500 mg PO 4–6 hr. for H/A (headache) would be administered to the patient every 4 to 6 hours when he or she complained of a headache. This order is a standing PRN order. p. 242

NOTES

78. *Lomotil tab 1 PO qid until diarrhea subsides* is which of the following types of order?
    a. Short order series
    b. Standing
    c. Standing PRN
    d. One time

79. Newly written doctor's orders may be recognized by which of the following:
    a. The orders are signed off
    b. The chart is out of the rack
    c. The chart is flagged
    d. The chart is lying open on the counter

80. The process of writing data on the doctor's order sheet to indicate completion of transcription of a set of orders is called:
    a. Kardexing
    b. Flagging
    c. Requisitioning
    d. Signing off

81. When arriving back to the nursing unit from lunch break, you find seven charts lying about the counter. You would:
    a. Read all of the orders, fax all of the pharmacy copies (document; faxed with date, time and initials), order all stat orders, give a copy of the orders to each patient's nurse, and then proceed to transcribe all other orders one chart at a time
    b. Proceed to transcribe orders using time written to establish priority, fax pharmacy copies and order stat orders, and give copies to nurses as you get to each chart
    c. Call the nurse manager for help
    d. Read all of the orders, transcribe all of the stat orders, proceed to transcribe orders one chart at a time, and fax pharmacy copies and all of the other necessary steps of transcription as you get to each chart

82. POCT would include which of the following procedures?
    a. KUB
    b. Spirometry
    c. Coombs test
    d. Glucose monitoring

83. Which of the following medications would be important to note when ordering an ABG?
    a. Lasix
    b. Demerol
    c. warfarin
    d. vancomycin

84. An order for "cl liq, adv DAT" would give the patient's nurse the option of ordering which of the following diets for the patient:
    a. 2.5 gm sodium
    b. 1000 cal ADA
    c. Mech soft
    d. Low cholesterol

85. Which of the following is a brand name for a feeding pump?
    a. I-med
    b. Accu-chek
    c. Guaiac
    d. Kangaroo

86. A feeding tube inserted into the an artificial opening into the abdominal wall extending into the stomach is called:
    a. Nasogastric feeding
    b. Total parenteral nutrition
    c. Gastrostomy feeding
    d. Gavage feeding

87. An order for knee-high Teds would require the health unit coordinator to:
    a. Order the Teds from the CSD as written
    b. Go into the patient's room to measure their legs
    c. Ask the patient over the intercom what size they would need
    d. Ask the patient's nurse to measure the patient for the Teds

88. A patient admitted with a diagnosis of a "pneumothorax" would most likely have an order written for the following equipment:
    a. Pleur-Evac
    b. Foot board
    c. K-pad
    d. Irrigation tray

78. **(a)** *Lomotil tab 1 PO qid until diarrhea subsides* would be administered four times a day until the patient's diarrhea goes away. This order would be a short order series. pp. 178, 240

79. **(c)** One way that newly written doctors' orders may be recognized is by the chart being flagged (usually by the doctor writing the order). pp. 160, 161

80. **(d)** Signing off by writing the full date, military time, and your full signature indicates the completion of transcription of a set of orders. The sign off is usually written one line below the physician's signature. pp. 166, 167

81. **(a)** Read all of the orders, fax all of the pharmacy copies (document: faxed with date, time, and initials), order all stat orders, give copy of orders to patient's nurse, and then proceed to transcribe all other orders one chart at a time. pp. 102, 103

82. **(d)** Glucose monitoring would be a POCT (point of care test) that would be performed at the bedside. p. 269

83. **(c)** Warfarin is the generic name for Coumadin, and would be important to note when ordering an ABG (arterial blood gas). pp. 250, 324

84. **(c)** *Mech soft* is a consistency diet that may be ordered by the patient's nurse when the doctor writes an order for DAT (diet as tolerated). p. 218

85. **(d)** A Kangaroo pump is a brand name for a feeding pump. p. 214

86. **(c)** A feeding tube inserted into the abdominal wall extending into the stomach is called a *gastrostomy feeding*. "gastr" is a word root meaning *stomach* and "stomy" is a suffix meaning *creation of an artificial opening*. pp. 221, 526

87. **(d)** When ordering Ted hose, the health unit coordinator would need to ask the patient's nurse to measure the patient for the Teds. p. 207

88. **(a)** A Pleur-Evac would be used for a patient admitted with a pneumothorax to release the air from the pleural cavity and re-expand the lung. pp. 204, 541

NOTES

89. Which of the following laboratory tests would likely be ordered on a daily basis when a patient is receiving TPN?
a. CBC
b. PT
c. CMP
d. ESR

90. A 2 hr PPBS would be ordered from which of the following laboratory divisions?
a. Hematology
b. Chemistry
c. Microbiology
d. Serology

91. A "BUN" is performed to diagnose a problem with which of the following organs:
a. Lung
b. Kidney
c. Esophagus
d. Pancreas

92. Which of the following diagnostic imaging procedures would require the patient to receive a bowel prep (cathartic):
a. KUB
b. CT of LS Spine
c. US of pelvis
d. BE

93. Which of the following diagnostic procedures would the health unit coordinator schedule to be performed last:
a. Sigmoidoscopy
b. Barium enema
c. Bone scan
d. KUB

94. An RN who acts as a liaison between the patient, the doctor, and the insurance company, and who coordinates the care for the hospitalized patient is called a:
a. Nurse coordinator
b. Nurse manager
c. Case manager
d. Vice president of nursing

95. Before a discharged patient leaves the hospital, the health unit coordinator should:
a. Go into the patient's room to check for any items left by the patient
b. Ask the patient to fill out an evaluation form regarding his or her hospitalization
c. Read the discharge order to make sure it doesn't include an order to be carried out before discharge
d. Make sure the patient has someone to ride home with

96. A doctor's order for isolation would require the health unit coordinator to order a/an:
a. Shroud from CSD
b. Isolation pack from CSD
c. Consult with the infectious disease doctor
d. Isolation specialist to care for the patient

97. A patient admitted with *osteogenic carcinoma* would be admitted to which of the following nursing units:
a. Oncology
b. Telemetry
c. Orthopedics
d. Pulmonary

98. Death of body tissue caused by lack of blood supply to an area of the body is called:
a. An abscess
b. Gangrene
c. A laceration
d. A 1st-degree burn

99. Another name for a CVA is a:
a. Seizure
b. Brain tumor
c. Stroke
d. Heart attack

100. The meninges are made up of three layers of connective tissue that surround the:
a. Abdominal muscles
b. Brain and spinal cord
c. Lung
d. Uterus

☑ ANSWERS AND RATIONALE

89. **(c)**   A CMP (comprehensive metabolic panel) would be ordered for a patient receiving TPN (total parenteral nutrition). p. 273

90. **(b)**   A 2-hour postprandial blood sugar would be ordered from the chemistry department to be drawn 2 hours after the patient finishes eating a meal. p. 274

91. **(b)**   A BUN (blood urea nitrogen) is a blood test performed in the chemistry division of the laboratory to diagnose a problem with the kidney. p. 273

92. **(d)**   A barium enema (BE) would require the patient to receive a bowel prep (cathartic) so the view of the colon is not obscured by fecal material. p. 297

93. **(b)**   A barium enema (BE) would be scheduled last, because this test uses barium, a medium that would obscure the view during the other procedures. p. 295

94. **(c)**   A case manager acts as a liaison between the patient, doctor, and the insurance company, and coordinates the patient's care while he or she is hospitalized. p. 22

95. **(c)**   The health unit coordinator should read the discharge order to make sure it doesn't include an order to be carried out before discharge. Often the doctor will leave a written prescription for the patient to take home in the chart as well. p. 396

96. **(b)**   An isolation pack including gowns and masks is required when an isolation order is written by the doctor. p. 432

97. **(a)**   A patient admitted with osteogenic carcinoma (cancerous tumor originating in the bone) would be admitted to the oncology unit. pp. 457, 459, 472

98. **(b)**   Gangrene occurs when there is a lack of blood supply to an area of the body, causing death of body tissue. pp. 452, 453

99. **(c)**   A CVA (cerebral vascular accident) is commonly known as a stroke. p. 482

100. **(b)**   The meninges are made up of three layers of connective tissue that surround the brain and spinal cord. p. 482

NOTES

101. An instrument used to view the eye is called a/an:
    a. Otoscope
    b. Opthalmoscope
    c. Sigmoidoscope
    d. Ophthalmoscope

102. A needle puncture into the pleural space in the chest cavity to remove pleural fluid for diagnostic or therapeutic reasons would require the health unit coordinator to prepare a consent for a/an:
    a. Thoracentesis
    b. Sternal puncture
    c. Endoscopy
    d. Amniocentesis

103. A patient admitted to the hospital with meningitis would have inflammation of the:
    a. Lining of the bowels
    b. Inner lining of the uterus
    c. Membranes of the spinal cord or brain
    d. Inner lining of the eye

104. A patient admitted to the hospital with a diagnosis of Alzheimer's disease would be admitted to which of the following hospital units?
    a. Oncology
    b. Surgery
    c. Neurology
    d. Pulmonary

105. A sigmoidoscopy would be performed in which of the following hospital departments?
    a. Surgery
    b. Endoscopy
    c. Treatment room
    d. Diagnostic Imaging

106. A patient's biopsy report states that the specimen is *malignant*. This means that the patient has:
    a. A build up of metal in his or her blood
    b. Cancer that will become progressively worse
    c. Cancer that is in remission
    d. An absence of cancer

107. A patient's biopsy report states the specimen is *benign*. This means that the patient has:
    a. Cancer that is spreading
    b. An absence of cancer
    c. Infection
    d. A malignancy

108. In the order, *call hospitalist if temp > 101 °*, the symbol ">" indicates:
    a. Exactly
    b. Less than
    c. Greater than
    d. Equal to

109. A patient scheduled for a surgical procedure called a *CABG* would have a diagnosis of:
    a. Varicose veins
    b. Fractured vertebrae caused by a car accident
    c. Occlusion or narrowing of the coronary arteries
    d. Cerebrovascular accident

110. Which of the following doctors' orders would instruct occupational therapy to assist the patient to return to the greatest possible functional independence?
    a. ABR
    b. CBG
    c. ADL
    d. BSC

111. A doctor's order for a *CMP* would be sent to which of the following hospital departments?
    a. Physical Therapy
    b. Occupational Therapy
    c. Laboratory
    d. Diagnostic Imaging

112. An order for an *EGD* would be sent to which of the following hospital departments?
    a. Endoscopy
    b. Surgery
    c. Diagnostic Imaging
    d. Laboratory

ANSWERS AND RATIONALE

101. **(d)** An ophthalmoscope is an instrument used to view the eye. Ophthalmoscope is often misspelled. p. 500

102. **(a)** A thoracentesis is a procedure performed by a needle puncture into the pleural space in the chest cavity to remove pleural fluid. This procedure does require a signed consent. p. 367

103. **(c)** A patient admitted with meningitis would have inflammation of the membranes of the spinal cord or brain. p. 488

104. **(c)** A patient admitted with Alzheimer's disease would be admitted to the neurology department. pp. 34, 483

105. **(b)** A sigmoidoscopy (visual examination of the sigmoid colon) would be performed in the endoscopy department. p. 321

106. **(b)** Cancer that will become progressively worse. p. 452

107. **(b)** An absence of cancer. p. 452

108. **(c)** The symbol ">" means *greater than*. p. 332

109. **(c)** The patient would have an occlusion or narrowing of the coronary arteries called *coronary artery disease (CAD)*. The procedure is called a *coronary artery bypass graft (CABG)*. p. 507

110. **(c)** ADL (activities of daily living) is an order that would instruct occupational therapy to assist the patient to return to the greatest possible functional independence. pp. 331, 346

111. **(c)** CMP (comprehensive metabolic panel) is a blood test consisting of a series of chemistries performed in the chemistry division of the laboratory. p. 273

112. **(a)** An order for an EGD (esophagogastroduodenoscopy) would be performed in the endoscopy department. pp. 313, 320

NOTES

113. An order for the patient to receive *SVN treatments* would be sent to which of the following departments?
    a. Physical Therapy
    b. Occupational Therapy
    c. Radiation
    d. Respiratory Care

114. Which of the following orders would require the health unit coordinator to prepare a consent form?
    a. PICC
    b. TPN
    c. TCDB
    d. IV

115. You have received a poor yearly evaluation. The nurse manager said that your performance was unsatisfactory. Your best response would be:
    a. Tell her she is not being fair and you deserve better
    b. Ask for specifics regarding your unsatisfactory performance and for suggestions for improvement
    c. Threaten to quit if she does not give you a better evaluation and tell her that you will file a grievance
    d. Remind her of all the positive things you have accomplished, in-services you have attended, and tell her that everyone else thinks you are doing a great job.

116. You don't feel that your job is challenging and would like to apply for a management job that will soon be available on the nursing unit where you work. The best way to be considered for the position is to:
    a. Be especially nice to the nurse manager who will be interviewing candidates for the position
    b. Ask all the nurses on the unit to put in a good word for you to the nurse manager
    c. Perform your usual tasks to the best of your ability and volunteer to work on committees when possible
    d. Remind the nurse manager of any faults that the other candidates may have

117. Which of the following indicates proper telephone etiquette when placing a caller on hold?
    a. "I'm placing you on hold now."
    b. "Hold please."
    c. Say nothing and place the caller on hold
    d. "May I place you on hold?"

118. To correct a series of errors on the graphic record, you would:
    a. Cross through each of them and write in correct information
    b. Ask the nurse to make the corrections on the record
    c. Recopy the graphic record, using the correct data
    d. White out the incorrect entries and write in correct information

119. You realize that you ordered a laboratory test on the wrong patient after the test was performed. You should:
    a. Order the test on the correct patient and say nothing
    b. Call the nurse manager and ask what to do
    c. Advise the patients involved, notify both patients nurses, and complete an incident report
    d. Order the test on the correct patient, notify the patients' nurses, and complete an incident report

120. Which of the following best describes *listening with empathy?*
    a. Showing a lot of patience and tolerance while someone is talking
    b. Demonstrating sympathy
    c. Listening only to what interests you
    d. Listening with both the heart and mind to understand

☑ *ANSWERS AND RATIONALE*

113. **(d)** An SVN (small volume nebulizer) would be sent to the respiratory care department. pp. 331, 340

114. **(a)** A PICC (peripherally inserted central catheter) would require the health unit coordinator to prepare a consent form. p. 197

115. **(b)** Ask for specifics regarding your unsatisfactory performance and for suggestions to improve. The process should provide both positive feedback and also suggestions on how to improve in areas where improvement is needed. p. 86

116. **(c)** Perform your usual tasks to the best of your ability and volunteer to work on committees when possible. p. 82

117. **(d)** Proper telephone etiquette when placing a caller on hold is to ask if you may place the caller on hold and wait for an answer. pp. 45, 46

118. **(c)** To correct a series of errors on a patient's graphic record, you would recopy the graphic record using the correct data. A line would be marked across the incorrect graphic record, and a notation stating "recopied" with the date and your initials, would be placed on both graphic records. Both graphic records would be placed in the patient's chart. p. 416

119. **(d)** Order the test on the correct patient, notify the patients' nurses, and complete an incident report. pp. 106, 107

120. **(d)** Listening with empathy is listening with both the heart and mind to understand. p. 64

NOTES